Mindfulness-Based Relapse Prevention for Addictive Behaviors

Also Available

Assessment of Addictive Behaviors, Second Edition
Edited by Dennis M. Donovan and G. Alan Marlatt

Brief Alcohol Screening and Intervention for College Students (BASICS):
A Harm Reduction Approach
Linda A. Dimeff, John S. Baer, Daniel R. Kivlahan, and G. Alan Marlatt

Harm Reduction:
Pragmatic Strategies for Managing High-Risk Behaviors, Second Edition
Edited by G. Alan Marlatt, Mary E. Larimer, and Katie Witkiewitz

Relapse Prevention: Maintenance Strategies in the Treatment
of Addictive Behaviors, Second Edition
Edited by G. Alan Marlatt and Dennis M. Donovan

Mindfulness-Based Relapse Prevention for Addictive Behaviors

A Clinician's Guide

SECOND EDITION

Sarah Bowen, Neha Chawla,
Joel Grow, and G. Alan Marlatt

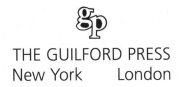

THE GUILFORD PRESS
New York   London

See page 204 for terms of use for audio files.

The authors have checked with sources believed to be reliable in their efforts to provide
information that is complete and generally in accord with the standards of practice that are
accepted at the time of publication. However, in view of the possibility of human error or changes
in behavioral, mental health, or medical sciences, neither the authors, nor the editor and publisher,
nor any other party who has been involved in the preparation or publication of this work warrants
that the information contained herein is in every respect accurate or complete, and they are not
responsible for any errors or omissions or the results obtained from the use of such information.
Readers are encouraged to confirm the information contained in this book with other sources.

Library of Congress Cataloging-in-Publication Data is available from the publisher.

ISBN 978-1-4625-4531-5 (paperback) — ISBN 978-1-4625-4532-2 (hardcover)

About the Authors

Sarah Bowen, PhD, a clinical psychologist, is Associate Professor at Pacific University in Portland, Oregon. She is a longtime Research Fellow with the Mind and Life Institute and Trainer at the Center for Mindfulness at the University of California, San Diego. Dr. Bowen specializes in mindfulness-based approaches for treatment of addictive behaviors. Her research and more than 50 publications have focused on mechanisms of change and on treatment adaptations to best serve diverse populations and settings, with particular interests in dual diagnosis and underserved communities. Dr. Bowen facilitates and supervises mindfulness-based relapse prevention (MBRP) groups in numerous settings, including private and county treatment agencies, medical centers, and prisons. She presents, consults, and provides instruction internationally.

Neha Chawla, PhD, a clinical psychologist, is founder and Director of the Seattle Mindfulness Center. In her private psychotherapy practice, Dr. Chawla provides empirically supported mindfulness- and acceptance-based treatments and facilitates MBRP groups. A co-developer of MBRP, she serves on the clinical faculty of the Department of Psychology at the University of Washington. Dr. Chawla has written on a variety of topics related to mindfulness and has been involved in research on issues related to therapist training and competence. She has facilitated groups in both private and community settings and has conducted numerous therapist training workshops in the United States and internationally.

Joel Grow, PhD, is a clinical psychologist at the Seattle Mindfulness Center and serves on the clinical faculty of the Department of Psychology at the University of Washington. He provides evidence-supported treatment that incorporates self-compassion, mindfulness, and acceptance-based approaches. Dr. Grow was a member of the University of Washington research team that developed MBRP, and he remains active in MBRP delivery, training, and evaluation. He has provided behavioral health care and led workshops in a range of private and community settings. Dr. Grow co-developed and served as lead instructor for a 9-month certificate program at the University of Washington, where he received the UW Award for Teaching Excellence.

G. Alan Marlatt, PhD, until his death in 2011, was Director of the Addictive Behaviors Research Center and Professor of Psychology at the University of Washington. For over 30 years, Dr. Marlatt conducted pioneering work on understanding and preventing relapse in substance abuse treatment and was a leading proponent of the harm reduction approach to treating addictive behaviors. He was a recipient of honors including the Jellinek Memorial Award for outstanding contributions to knowledge in the field of alcohol studies, the Robert Wood Johnson Foundation's Innovators Combating Substance Abuse Award, the Research Society on Alcoholism's Distinguished Researcher Award, and the Career/Lifetime Achievement Award from the Association for Behavioral and Cognitive Therapies.

Preface

Mindfulness-based relapse prevention (MBRP) is a program integrating mindfulness meditation practices with traditional relapse prevention (RP). Traditional RP is a cognitive-behavioral intervention designed to help prevent or manage relapse following treatment for addictive behaviors. Similarly, MBRP was originally designed as an outpatient aftercare program to support maintenance of treatment gains and foster a sustainable lifestyle for individuals in recovery. In this second edition of *Mindfulness-Based Relapse Prevention for Addictive Behaviors,* we offer an updated program designed to target primary risk factors for relapse, including deep-seated beliefs, mental and behavioral habits, and urges and cravings common to a variety of addictive behaviors.

This work originated at the Addictive Behaviors Research Center at the University of Washington in the early 2000s with an intention to integrate evidence-based programs and best practices into addictions treatment. Dr. G. Alan Marlatt, who founded and directed the center, passed away in 2011. He was a mentor to the other three authors of this edition, and his legacy and impact in the addictions field are immeasurable.

Joel Grow joins us for this second edition. As did the other two authors, Dr. Grow began his career as a graduate student in Dr. Marlatt's research lab. This book represents the culmination of over a decade of facilitating, training in, and studying the MBRP program, as we have carried on Dr. Marlatt's work and brought our own research and clinical discoveries to the program. Our hope is that this offering is of true benefit to readers and those they serve.

In practice, we have found MBRP to be effective as a stand-alone aftercare program as well as a support to other programs, such as Alcoholics Anonymous and Narcotics Anonymous. For some, MBRP may complement these other programs, whereas for others, MBRP may offer a helpful alternative. Clients are invited to find how this best fits into their lives, beliefs, and circumstances, and to use the practices and skills offered to create a path to recovery that is most viable for them. In that vein, MBRP is also consistent with a harm reduction approach that allows clients to connect with their own motivation and to cultivate compassion for wherever they may be on their journey.

Similarly, we have found the program to be appropriate not only for individuals with substance use disorders, but for those with a broad array of addictive behaviors, and it can reinforce diverse treatment objectives, supporting but not requiring a specific goal. This approach allows individuals to learn for themselves what brings about their suffering, what freedom from suffering means for them, and how to find their own path out of the trappings of addictive behaviors.

Acknowledgments

We are tremendously grateful to the countless teachers, colleagues, and friends who have offered collaboration, support, talent, and wisdom to the creation of this program. For their steady support and inspiration, and for the daily opportunities for practice, we would like to thank our families, partners, and friends. For their seemingly endless wisdom and compassionate hearts, we are deeply grateful to the meditation teachers whose offerings have inspired us and helped us deepen our own experience and understanding. For their enthusiasm and fresh perspectives, we thank our students and trainees. Finally, for their faith, commitment, and practice, we are immensely grateful to all of the participants in our MBRP groups.

The structure and content of MBRP are largely inspired by and based on the work of Jon Kabat-Zinn and colleagues at the Center for Mindfulness in Medicine, Health Care, and Society at the University of Massachusetts Medical School and the seminal work of Kabat-Zinn's mindfulness-based stress reduction program, as described in his book *Full Catastrophe Living* (1990). Additionally, several exercises are derived or adapted from the work of Zindel Segal, Mark Williams, and John Teasdale in *Mindfulness-Based Cognitive Therapy for Depression* (2nd ed.; 2013).

The Addictive Behaviors Research Center's Mindfulness-Based Relapse Prevention Treatment Development Project was funded by National Institute on Drug Abuse Grants No. 1 R21 DA019562-01A1, G. Alan Marlatt, PhD, Principal Investigator, and 1 R01 DA025764-01A1, G. Alan Marlatt, PhD, and Sarah Bowen, PhD, Principal Investigators.

Contents

Introduction   1

PART I   **Foundations and Framework**   5

PART II   **Facilitator's Guide**   29

SESSION 1   Automatic Pilot and Mindful Awareness   33

SESSION 2   A New Relationship with Discomfort   52

SESSION 3   From Reacting to Responding   75

SESSION 4   Mindfulness in Challenging Situations   95

SESSION 5   Acceptance and Skillful Action   112

SESSION 6   Seeing Thoughts as Thoughts   128

SESSION 7   Supporting and Sustaining Well-Being   145

SESSION 8   Social Support and Continuing Practice   158

PART III   **Research and Adaptations**   *171*

APPENDIX   *185*

REFERENCES   *195*

INDEX   *199*

LIST OF AUDIO TRACKS   *204*

Introduction

We suspect that clinicians drawn to this program have significant interest in or experience with both mindfulness practice and the treatment of addictive behaviors. Perhaps, similar to many of your clients, you are seeking an alternative approach to or a fresh perspective on addictive behavior and relapse. Maybe you are seeking another means of helping clients find freedom from the destructive cycle of harmful behaviors. It is a similar search that led us to the development of MBRP. It has been our intention to bring practices of mindful awareness to individuals suffering from addiction. The practices in this program are designed to foster increased awareness of triggers and the habitual or "automatic" reactions that seem to control many of our lives. These practices help cultivate the ability to pause, observe present experience, and bring awareness to the range of choices before each of us in every moment. Ultimately, we are working toward freedom from deeply ingrained and often catastrophic patterns of thought and behavior.

This approach represents a culmination of our combined experiences with treating and researching substance use disorder. It also represents our personal journeys with meditation practice and the desire to offer to others what has been so valuable in our own lives. It is through the inspiration and support of those who have pioneered mindfulness-based programs that this program first came to fruition and has continued to grow in impact. Our mentor, Dr. Alan Marlatt, set the stage for this work with his contributions to the field of relapse prevention (particularly cognitive-behavioral treatments for addictive behaviors), his advocacy for a harm reduction approach, and his interest in meditation. His work, along with the work of others who have pioneered mindfulness-based programs, has provided a platform for us to integrate existing knowledge and frameworks with what we have learned from our own research, practice, and personal journeys with meditation.

We cannot overemphasize the importance of personal meditation practice as the basis for training and preparation. Although MBRP is also informed by principles of cognitive and behavioral psychology, mindfulness practice is what differentiates this program from many other substance abuse treatments. Our hope is that, in the tradition of mindfulness-based stress reduction (MBSR) and mindfulness-based cognitive therapy (MBCT), this program will remain grounded in mindfulness meditation. Familiarity and experience with cognitive therapy, facilitation of groups, and work with addictions is ideal, but perhaps secondary to a foundation of personal mindfulness practice. It is their own practice that allows MBRP facilitators to model the attitudes and behaviors that they are inviting participants to cultivate and that are at the heart of the program. When first developing this program, we learned that there were simply no shortcuts, and a decade later, we continue to observe this; it is only through personal practice, and the experience of the challenges and insights that come with it, that we as facilitators can truly begin to embody the qualities MBRP is intended to foster.

For those who may be new to mindfulness practice, we encourage personal exploration of mindfulness meditation before embarking upon delivery of this treatment. As a starting point, you might explore the meditation resources listed in the final session of the program. In addition to the books and audio recordings listed, we highly recommend direct instruction from an experienced teacher and participation in at least one intensive meditation retreat. Training in the insight, or vipassana, meditation tradition is most consistent with the practices included in this program.

Originally published in 2010, this guide has served as a foundation for countless MBRP groups and professional training workshops in the United States and abroad. We have continued to study, refine, deliver, and evaluate the program. Over a decade has passed since the original version of this guide, and throughout that time, both research and clinical experience have enriched the treatment protocol in several ways. Thus, this second edition retains the foundational aspects of an integrated science-informed clinical approach, while being informed by advances in the field.

In this second edition, we offer several updated materials. The main focus of the program and of each session is consistent with the original version, but select practices and exercises have been revised and new practices added. We now provide easier access to printable PDFs of worksheets, as well as links to recordings of all MBRP practices to use in whatever ways best support the program.

The guide is organized in three main sections. Part I lays out the background and foundation for the development of MBRP and offers a discussion of our experience with and recommendations for facilitating the treatment. This includes examples of challenges encountered, lessons learned, and issues requiring further consideration.

As part of the new edition, we also include an updated summary of supporting research. The body of scientific literature on both addictive behaviors and mindfulness-based approaches has advanced markedly over the past decade, and research on MBRP has similarly progressed. This growth has resulted in a clearer understanding of neural and behavioral processes underlying addictive behaviors, as well as mechanisms of change in mindfulness-based approaches. This has deepened our understanding of how mindfulness practice can directly target factors that initiate and perpetuate addictive behaviors.

Part II offers a session-by-session guide to support MBRP clinicians delivering of the program. These chapters provide a detailed discussion of the themes and practices included in each session, common experiences encountered by MBRP participants, and issues or challenges that may arise. They also list materials needed, provide a structure and outline, and include worksheets, handouts, and examples of the guided meditation practices. The 8-week structure includes three basic sections. The first three sessions focus on practicing mindful awareness and integrating mindfulness practices into both challenging situations and daily life. The next three sessions emphasize acceptance of present experience and application of mindfulness practices to behavioral patterns and relapse prevention, and the final two sessions expand to include issues of self-care, support networks, and sustaining well-being. Each session is designed to build on the previous one, and sessions are intended to be practiced in the order in which we describe them here. The structure offered in this program, in combination with the facilitator's personal daily mindfulness practice, offers clients new perspectives and skills to guide them not only in the day-to-day challenges of recovery but also in the moment-to-moment awareness, compassion, and freedom that mindfulness practice can bring.

The newly added Part III offers a brief overview of other advancements in our own work and in the broader field, focusing on more sensitive and effective cultural adaptations, diverse contexts in which the program is offered, and more complex individual psychological profiles. It includes alternative formats of the program, such as a rolling group model, and a 6-week versus 8-week structure. Having developed this program over a decade ago, we have also seen significant changes in technology. When the original program was created, for example, smartphones were brand new, mobile apps hadn't taken off yet, and web-based distribution of meditation instruction audio files was rare. In Part III, we discuss how these changes in technology can offer supplemental support to participants as they move through the program.

PART I

Foundations and Framework

From the outset we envisioned MBRP as an integration of standard cognitive-behavioral-based relapse prevention treatment with mindfulness meditation practices. Thus, the MBRP curriculum includes identification of personal triggers and situations in which participants are particularly vulnerable, along with practical skills to use in such times. Alongside these skills, participants learn mindfulness practices designed to heighten awareness of and shift the relationship to all experience, both internal (emotions, thoughts, sensations) and external (environmental cues), promoting a greater sense of choice, compassion, and freedom. The program is informed by MBSR (Kabat-Zinn, 1990), MBCT (Segal, Williams, & Teasdale, 2013), and Daley and Marlatt's (2006) relapse prevention protocol.

In the following pages, we place the program in its larger context, highlight core intentions, and describe our experiences developing and facilitating it. We offer our experience and ideas regarding selecting and training MBRP facilitators, conducting MBRP groups, and navigating logistical, theoretical, and clinical issues that may arise. Just as we have benefited immensely from the experience and advice of our MBSR and MBCT mentors, it is our hope that our experiences might be useful to those embarking upon a similar journey.

CHANGES IN THE FIELD OF ADDICTION

In many ways, we are in a different time scientifically and culturally than when the first edition of this guide was written. The field has seen several changes in defining and understanding addiction.

A significant shift occurred with the publication of the fifth edition of the *Diagnostic and Statistical Manual of Mental Disorders* (DSM-5; American Psychiatric Association, 2013), which describes addictive behaviors on a spectrum of severity, rather than as consisting of discrete categories. DSM-5 also now includes other addictive behaviors, such as gambling, in its diagnostic lexicon. This revised model reflects the underlying commonalities across addictive behaviors, and the continuum-based framework supports a more functional/contextual approach. Our work has followed a parallel evolution, with a better understanding of mechanisms underlying addictive behavior cycles and practices designed to highlight and address these mechanisms and functions of behavior. A functional analysis of behavior recognizes that people typically engage in a behavior repeatedly because it serves an underlying purpose or function (O'Neill et al., 1997). In addictive behaviors, one person may engage in a behavior to avoid or soothe pain, while another may do so to seek pleasure, or to avoid embarrassment in a social situation. The field of addiction and its treatment increasingly recognizes these functional similarities across addictive behaviors, including urges, cravings, and emotional dysregulation; reduced negative affect and increased positive affect as a result of engaging in the behavior; and similar activation in the brain's reward circuitry.

The MBRP model similarly views addictive behaviors on a continuum, versus as a discrete condition, and as serving a specific function, which may vary between individuals. The program thus includes practices to develop awareness of these underlying functions and targets underlying mechanisms, including craving and tolerance of challenging emotional and physical experiences.

THE SOCIOPOLITICAL CONTEXT OF ADDICTION AND MINDFULNESS-BASED TREATMENTS

Alongside changes in the addiction field are changes in mindfulness-based treatment approaches and in the larger sociopolitical landscape. Most current definitions of addiction position the behavior in an individualistic framework that emphasizes personal action and internal mechanisms, and this book is no exception, as we describe an intervention model that emphasizes individual freedom and choice. However, we acknowledge the importance of viewing this model within current trends in mindfulness-based treatments and the larger cultural and sociopolitical context of addictive behaviors.

The field of addiction and addictions treatment has long been fraught with inequity and injustice. Race and economic inequalities have a significant impact on substance use, access to treatment, and treatment outcomes, as well as legal, social, and political ramifications, all of which feed into a system of oppression woven into the fabric of U.S. society. Other countries in which this program is being adapted and implemented may have their own manifestations of these injustices.

In the United States, these inequities are reflected in policies that often view addiction as a failure of personal responsibility and characteristic of a culture of poverty (i.e., cultural norms counter to societal norms of hard work and lawfulness; Powell, 2012), and downplay the impact of systemic inequality, politics, and racism. This is perhaps most evident in the criminal justice system, which historically has taken a "zero tolerance" approach and declared war on people with substance use problems. People of color are arrested and convicted at higher rates than whites and receive more severe sentencing for similar offenses (Bureau of Justice Statistics, 2018). Some of these prejudices and assumptions seep into treatment environments as well, resulting in a punitive extension of the criminal justice system and further perpetuating experiences of institutional oppression. These trends are linked to lower rates of treatment seeking and completion (Chartier & Caetano, 2010; Guerrero, 2013), as well as poorer treatment outcomes (Blume, 2016; Blume, Lovato, Thyken, & Denny, 2012) in people of color. We hope that MBRP can offer an inclusive, just, and nonpunitive approach that emphasizes trust in and respect for each individual's experience.

Mindfulness-based treatments and their applications have increased dramatically, as has the popularity of mindfulness in the mainstream culture. This is evident in both the scientific research and in popular media. While this may support increased accessibility and engagement, it also presents some challenges. These include frequent use of the term "mindfulness" without a clear understanding of what it refers to or the practices involved in its cultivation, and a misconception of mindfulness as a state of bliss or magical panacea for everything that ails us.

Further, most mindfulness-based programs were created, and frequently delivered by, white facilitators. While this is changing, the bulk of the research on mindfulness and mindfulness-based interventions was at least initially based on white participants (Amaro, Spear, Vallejo, Conron, & Black, 2014), and many current intervention models were initially developed within a largely white cultural context. This may have resulted in infusion of white-centric values, language, stories, cultural references, and assumptions.

Although the long-term effort involved in dismantling these internal and external structures is beyond the scope of this treatment guide, recognizing and acknowledging these influences and potential is essential. As facilitators coming from any cultural or racial background, there are a few things we might keep in mind. While we may aspire to create a space where all feel welcome, societal imbalances may seep into our language in insidious ways. For instance, a seemingly benign statement such as "all of our minds work similarly" may be liberating to some, but may be experienced as deeply invalidating for those who already feel unseen or different. Messages that practice is a way to reduce suffering may imply that we are all responsible for our own suffering and freedom, concealing the role of institutionalized systems of oppression. This may be of particular relevance for facilitators who are coming from a place of privilege.

Engaging in and deepening our own mindfulness practice may help us become aware of our biases, observe our own conditioned patterns of thinking, feeling, and behaving, and help us begin to see and undo deep seated and potentially hurtful patterns of thought and action.

FACILITATING MBRP GROUPS

Ideally, an MBRP facilitator embodies curiosity and genuine interest in the present experience of participants, similar to the curiosity we cultivate in our own experiences in meditation practice. The facilitators view themselves as guides who use their own experience as a facilitation tool, rather than as experts or even teachers. Because facilitators encourage investigation and trust of one's own experience, the core principles of MBRP are elicited from participants whenever possible and are explored through experiential practices and *inquiry* (described below), rather than through "teaching." This encourages participants to see their own habits of mind and patterns of behavior and to discover what is true from observation of their own experience.

Structure

The structured protocol has session-by-session agendas containing practices and worksheets integrating principles from both cognitive-behavioral therapy (CBT) and traditional mindfulness teachings. Creativity and a shared curiosity, however, are what bring the program to life. Although the program is presented as eight distinct sessions, the content may need to be presented in alternate formats to fit specific contexts (see Part III). When making such modifications, an understanding of and adherence to the core intentions of the program and practices should remain at the forefront.

Core Intentions

1. **Increasing awareness** of our bodies, minds, and behaviors, including thoughts, emotional states, habit patterns, and reactions.

2. **Recognizing** and **interrupting automatic behavior**, creating the opportunity for agency and choice.

3. Learning a new way of **relating to discomfort**—with openness, curiosity, and acceptance, rather than aversion.

4. Cultivating **kindness and compassion** for the full range of our experiences.

Because teachers of mindfulness meditation encourage investigation and trust of one's own experience, the core principles of MBRP are elicited from participants whenever possible and are explored through experiential practices and inquiry. This encourages participants to see their own habits of mind and patterns of behavior and to discover what is true from observation of their own experience.

Inquiry

Both the style and the structure of groups are intended to emphasize each participant's direct experience, versus concepts or stories about our experiences. Thus, sessions typically begin with experiential exercises, followed by a period of brief discussion or "inquiry" (Segal et al., 2013). The intention is to keep these discussions centered on present experience, and at key points to relate that experience to relapse, recovery, craving, or lifestyle factors. Keeping inquiry focused on direct experience reflects a central intention of these mindfulness practices: to notice what is actually arising in the moment (or "direct experience") rather than getting lost in interpretations and stories. However, participants, especially in group treatment settings, are often accustomed to telling stories *about* their experience. Facilitators, too, are often in the habit of working with content or offering potential solutions. The process here is different. It requires facilitators to continually redirect interactions to exploration of the immediate, present experience (i.e., sensations in the body, thoughts, emotions or urges) versus the interpretation, analysis, or story about the experiences. When a participant begins discussing a story or concept, or evaluating his or her experience, just as in meditation practice itself, facilitators encourage "letting go and beginning again" by redirecting the participant to the experience in the present moment. The inquiry process itself thus becomes an example of the mind's tendency to veer off into thoughts and stories, and another practice in bringing focus back to present experience.

As illustrated in Figure 1.1 (adapted from MBCT), the inquiry process centers on differentiating between *direct experience* (often sensation, arising thought, or emotion) and *proliferations or reactions to* experience (e.g., stories, judgments). The observation of direct experience is the primary intention, and repeated discernment between the initial experience and reactions to it can be helpful in recognizing when our attention has been pulled away. These reactions or "add-ons" might be physical (such as tension or resistance), cognitive (such as proliferative thoughts or stories), or emotional (such as frustration or yearning) and may trigger further reactions. For example, there may be a primary experience, such as an intense physical sensation, followed by a thought about that experience, such as "I can't do this" and then an emotional reaction to the thought, such as a feeling of defeat. This proliferation might continue with another thought, such as "I knew I shouldn't have come to this group."

The inquiry process helps participants distinguish between an initial experience (e.g., physical sensation) and the thoughts or reactions that might follow it by encouraging them to repeatedly return their focus to what is actually occurring in the moment. With practice, participants begin to recognize when they are caught in stories or proliferations and realize they have the choice and ability to pause and return to present experience. Practicing this process of recognition and returning to the present, both in meditation practice and inquiry, strengthens our awareness and nonreactivity, alleviating some of the undue suffering our minds often cause.

The inquiry process may also highlight ways in which the experiences arising in meditation (both the direct experiences and our reactions to it) are familiar or unfamiliar. For example, a facilitator may inquire, "How is this similar to or different from what your mind usually does?" or "Have you noticed this about your mind before?" Facilitators may also ask how this experience is related to participants' lives (e.g., "How might what you just experienced be related to substance use or to relapse?"). This link between what is being experienced in the meditation and habitual patterns and behaviors may not be explicit in every interaction but is central to the overall purpose of the program (i.e., recognizing familiar or habitual patterns vs. unfamiliar or new ways of experiencing or relating to our experiences).

Finally, inquiry is intended to be an exploration of the shared tendencies of the mind rather than of any one individual's story. Highlighting that "this is what minds sometimes do" (e.g., wander off, ruminate) can help diminish the identification with this pattern and cultivate compassion. A facilitator might ask, "Does anyone else relate to this?" or "Isn't it interesting how minds sometimes do that?" to reaffirm that there are commonalities in how our minds work (see Figure I.1). However, we emphasize awareness and caution when making these statements to avoid unintentionally invalidating any individual's particular history or experience, particularly when it relates to being marginalized or feeling unseen (see "The Sociopolitical Context of Addiction and Mindfulness-Based Treatments," above).

Inquiry Framework

As illustrated in Figure I.1, the primary domains of inquiry are Awareness, Familiarity versus Newness, Relevance, and Common humanity. These elements are designed to help participants discern between, and notice effects of, direct experience versus reactions or stories about the experience. **Awareness** of raw or direct moment-to-moment experience is the most central of these elements. Facilitators explore this by, first and foremost, being curious about participants' experiences and helping them return repeatedly to a focus on what is occurring in the present (i.e., sensations, thoughts, emotions, urges) versus stories or interpretation that the

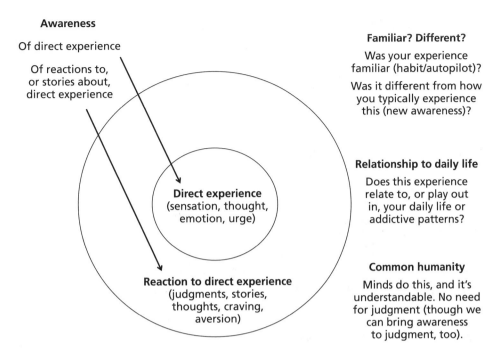

Awareness

Of direct experience

Of reactions to, or stories about, direct experience

Direct experience
(sensation, thought, emotion, urge)

Reaction to direct experience
(judgments, stories, thoughts, craving, aversion)

Familiar? Different?

Was your experience familiar (habit/autopilot)?

Was it different from how you typically experience this (new awareness)?

Relationship to daily life

Does this experience relate to, or play out in, your daily life or addictive patterns?

Common humanity

Minds do this, and it's understandable. No need for judgment (though we can bring awareness to judgment, too).

FIGURE I.1. Inquiry process. Based on personal communication with Zindel V. Segal (March 8, 2010).

mind adds on. Facilitators also inquire about **familiarity**, or whether an experience is a new awareness or part of a habitual "autopilot" or default pattern. Rather than lecturing about how or why this practice is important, MBRP takes a more humble stance, asking participants why, or if, a practice or experience is **relevant**, or related, to the larger context of their day-to-day life. Finally, to illustrate that these experiences are examples of **being human**, versus personal deficits, facilitators might inquire whether others in the room had similar experiences.

Below are examples of how a facilitator might integrate these different elements into inquiry with a participant:

Awareness

General: "I'm curious about what you all noticed during that practice." (We are careful not to use language that elicits an evaluation of the experience, such as "How did you do with that practice?," or to suggest a "right" answer in the question, such as "Was this easier than the first time you tried this practice?")

Focusing on direct experience (sensations, thoughts, emotions): "Did you notice that anywhere in the body?" "What did that feel like?" "Were there thoughts or a story associated with that?" "And then what happened?" "Do you still feel that now?" "What do you notice as you are talking now?"

Encouraging further exploration: "Can I ask you more about X?" "Did that experience change or stay the same?" "What else did you notice?"

Awareness of relationship to experience: "How did you relate to the experience? Did you notice any judgment?" "How was it to be with that experience? Did you have any kind of reaction?"

Familiar or Different

Autopilot or habit: "Is that a familiar pattern for you?" "Is this a pattern you see in other areas of your life?"

New awareness or different way of relating: "Was that different from how you typically experience this?" "Is that something you've noticed before?"

Related to Bigger Picture/Daily Life

Relationship to daily life: "Is what you just described related to your life? To addiction or recovery?"

Relevance: "Why do you think we do this practice in this group?"

Common Humanity

Framing as natural tendency versus pathology: "It's certainly understandable that we want to avoid experiences that are challenging or uncomfortable. We evolved this way to protect ourselves."

Normalizing: "Did anyone else have a similar experience? Different?" "I noticed my mind wandering during that practice, too."

Daily Practice

Specific daily practices are suggested each week, and each session includes a review of the previous week's daily practices. Facilitators should encourage integration of both formal and informal practice into daily life and emphasize its importance, while not inspiring self-blame and judgment. Discussing practice-related struggles with lightness, compassion, and curiosity is helpful; struggles with daily mindfulness practice do not indicate another failed attempt at change, but rather represent another opportunity to observe the tendencies of the mind. Approaching these discussions nonjudgmentally and with a sense of curiosity can help normalize common challenges, encouraging participants to view these, too, as part of practice and something to be curious about rather than as a problem or failure. Facilitators might model this by asking, "Is anyone experiencing difficulty with practice? What thoughts or feelings do you notice when you realize or disclose that you haven't practiced?"

In an effort to encourage practice, facilitators may have an urge to "sell" the merits of meditation. Such attempts at persuasion often result in skepticism, guilt, or resistance on the part of participants. As an alternative, gently guided discussions with open-ended questions (e.g., "How do you think these practices might be helpful for relapse prevention?" or "What might help you to practice more regularly?" or "What do you think would be doable or reasonable for you this coming week?") allow group members to generate their own reasons and motivations for practice, promoting increased engagement and decreased resistance. This style of discussion seems to be the most effective approach, engendering a more cooperative, client-centered environment.

We have also found it helpful to invite participants to set their own intentions for home practice, suggesting that, similar to strengthening a muscle, consistent, regular practice, even if brief, may be most useful in shifting deeply ingrained habits and patterns. Asking participants what is feasible for them, and emphasizing that *any* practice is more useful than no practice are all, may invite engagement without setting participants up for increased self-judgment.

Co-Facilitation

Support from a co-facilitator can provide added perspective and support in navigating the dynamics and challenges of MBRP facilitation. It is regrettably easy to revert to habitual styles or to slip into "teaching" or "instructing" rather than eliciting themes from the group. Especially in the beginning stages, co-facilitators learn from one another, offering different voices and styles, keeping each other adherent to the stance and core themes of the sessions, providing support, and balancing each other's skills, perspectives, and experiences. That said, we recognize that this is a more resource-intensive model, and it may not be feasible to have more than one facilitator. For clinicians facilitating by themselves, consultation with other facilitators or supervisors may provide some of the same benefits.

FACILITATORS: SELECTION, TRAINING, AND PERSONAL PRACTICE

To adequately guide the different aspects of the MBRP program, it is valuable for facilitators to have experience with treatment for addictive behaviors, as well as group facilitation. However, as we mentioned in the Introduction, perhaps most important is an understanding of and experience with mindfulness practice. A primary concern in developing MBRP and training facilitators has been differentiating the program from standard CBT-based relapse prevention. We were wary of creating a CBT-based treatment with the simple addition of mindfulness "exercises." Instead, our intention was to create a program grounded in mindfulness practice, with relapse prevention skills presented and practiced in a way that was consistent with a mindfulness approach. Throughout the inception, training, and facilitation of groups, we have kept facilitators' mindfulness practice at the core of the treatment. We believe this is what makes the program a unique offering to the treatment community. We provide more in-depth discussion of the role of the facilitator's personal practice later (see the section on the importance of personal practice).

Training

Preparation for facilitation of MBRP involves not only an established personal mindfulness practice, but formal training in the model. As with the facilitation of MBRP, we intend MBRP facilitator training to reflect the present-centered, non-judgmental, and accepting qualities cultivated by mindfulness practice itself. The aim is to meet whatever arises—among trainees and clients alike—with curiosity, equanimity, and compassion and with an experiential, present-centered focus. We have found this to be effective not only in creating a space that supports exploration and growth, but also in allowing a playful, open approach that brings both warmth and flexibility to the program.

The background and basic theory of relapse prevention, mindfulness meditation, and the blending of these practices are important pieces of the training of MBRP facilitators; however, the central focus is on experiential learning. Facilitator training can take a number of forms. For example, many facilitators have participated in 3-day workshops in which the theory and rationale are presented on the first evening, followed by 2 full days of guidance through the eight sessions of MBRP, with as many of the practices conducted in "real time" as possible. Following this initial intensive training, facilitators meet weekly to practice leading each session with one another, with input and supervision from the trainers. Similar to the MBRP treatment protocol, the practices and exercises precede discussions, with a significant part of each session spent on the meditations and exercises themselves. The intention is to keep the ideas and discussions simple, elaborating only in ways that would facilitate and enhance the practice itself. Trainees share questions and experiences regarding their own practice, including frustrations and barriers, such as making time in their busy schedules, persistent wandering of attention, self-doubt, restlessness, and sleepiness. These challenges are common to both facilitators and participants and are thus helpful to work with firsthand.

Other trainings are offered using a 5-day residential retreat-style format, allowing a deeper and richer experience of the program. Inspired by the MBCT training model, the format encourages trainees and facilitators to temporarily set aside the demands of their daily lives and immerse themselves in practicing together for these 5 days. The initial 2 days are spent guiding trainees through the exercises and practices of MBRP. The third day focuses on silent practice, followed by 2 days of trainees facilitating exercises in smaller groups, with feedback offered by both trainers and fellow trainees.

Finally, following these workshops, opportunities for trainees to observe or co-facilitate a full 8-week session guided by experienced MBRP facilitators will further enrich the training experience, and we strongly recommend this whenever possible.

Although these formats may not always be feasible, it is highly recommended that facilitators participate in experiential training and have a background of practice before guiding MBRP. This book provides an outline for the program but is in no way able to offer the level of understanding that comes from personal mindfulness practice, training in the model, observation of other facilitators, and supervision.

Importance of Personal Practice

Discussed above, but bearing repeating, perhaps the most crucial factor in facilitating MBRP is the facilitators' personal mindfulness meditation practice. Supporting others in the practice comes from one's own lived experience and history of having encountered similar struggles; it cannot come from simply "understanding" a treatment manual or attending a brief workshop.

Often therapists will attempt to start a meditation practice at the beginning of MBRP facilitator training. As any practitioner knows, however, consistent practice is a challenge and often takes months or even years to establish. Despite best intentions, facilitators newer to meditation often struggle with schedule constraints (i.e., allotting time for regular practice), expectations and misconceptions about mindfulness, and issues of discomfort, doubt, and self-judgment. Although these challenges are commonly experienced along the meditative journey, for practitioners who do not have the experience of an intensive retreat or support from a teacher or community, these experiences can be discouraging and difficult to navigate. We thus suggest that those who are new to this practice begin by referring to the resources listed in Session 8 or find similar resources, and participate in at least one residential retreat in the insight meditation, or vipassana, tradition.

Given the internal nature of the meditative process, it is often difficult even for experienced facilitators to assess an individual's experience and understanding of these practices. For those with a limited understanding of the nuances of practice, this may result in a restricted ability to respond skillfully to questions, doubts, and misconceptions raised by participants. For example, one of the most common concerns that arise in the first few sessions is the expectation that the practice is supposed to bring feelings of calm and peace, and that they are "doing it wrong" or it is "not working" if they find that the mind is distracted by thoughts, emotions, or challenging physical experiences. Facilitators with a strong personal practice may respond to such comments by drawing on their own experience for guidance, and they may be able to anticipate and explore challenges, even when participants are unable to articulate these issues themselves. As the following example illustrates, these facilitators often pick up on subtleties based on personal experience. (This and all subsequent dialogue was excerpted from MBRP sessions and edited for anonymity and clarity.)

> PARTICIPANT: I practiced with the audio meditation instructions every day, but I was only able to do it for about 10 minutes each time.
>
>> [At this point, a facilitator might validate the participant for practicing each day. Those with awareness of and familiarity with their own reactions during meditation may take the additional step of inquiring about what may have occurred for the participant at the end of the 10 minutes.]
>
> FACILITATOR: It isn't always easy to make space for something new in your life. I am curious to know what you noticed about your experience before you turned off the guided meditation.
>
> PARTICIPANT: I just wanted to get up and do other things.
>
> FACILITATOR: Was there restlessness? [Redirects to the first step in the inquiry process: awareness of the immediate physical, emotional, or cognitive experience.]
>
> PARTICIPANT: Yeah, exactly.
>
> FACILITATOR: What does restlessness feel like to you?
>
> PARTICIPANT: It was just a fidgety feeling, like it was hard to sit still and focus on the breath and the voice on the recording.
>
> FACILITATOR: Any particular place in your body where you sensed that, do you recall? [Continues to explore the immediate experience.]
>
> PARTICIPANT: In my hands definitely, and sort of all over.
>
> FACILITATOR: Hmm. What was the sensation in your hands, if you remember?
>
> PARTICIPANT: They were sort of tingling and twitchy.
>
> FACILITATOR: And do you remember your reaction to being restless? Were

there any thoughts about it? [Inquires about reactions to immediate experience.]

PARTICIPANT: Yeah, kind of. I felt a little ashamed that I couldn't sit for more than 10 minutes.

FACILITATOR: Okay, you noticed a feeling of shame. What about thoughts? Any thoughts that you remember? [Distinguishes between thoughts and emotions]

PARTICIPANT: I guess the thought that I couldn't do it anymore, that I had to get up.

FACILITATOR: Okay, feelings of restlessness in the hands and elsewhere in the body, an urge to get up and do things, and maybe a thought like "I can't do this. I have to get up," and some shame. [Highlights physical, emotional, and cognitive reactions.]

PARTICIPANT: Yeah, I felt like I should be able to sit for longer than 10 minutes.

FACILITATOR: So a thought, "I should be able to sit longer"? [Differentiates between thoughts and feeling.]

PARTICIPANT: Yeah, that was all happening.

FACILITATOR: What would it be like to just notice that experience, in the same way that we have been noticing the breath, to bring the same attention and curiosity to it, as just another experience occurring in the moment? Noticing what restlessness really feels like and noticing your reaction to it. And maybe seeing if you can soften around it a little, just allowing it to be there and just observing it, even for a moment? And then you may make the choice to get up or not.

In this dialogue, the facilitator is encouraging awareness of the physical, emotional, and cognitive components of experience, as well as urges that arise. She helps the participant recognize the initial experience and several reactions that followed. She is also modeling the curiosity, openness, and nonjudgmental stance that participants are asked to have toward themselves in relation to whatever arises, both during and in relation to the meditation practice. Notice, too, that she does not shift into problem solving (e.g., suggestions for how the participant might practice for longer periods of time).

Without the personal experience of having navigated one's own internal world in this way, facilitators might not respond with the same level of awareness, curiosity, and acceptance. Facilitators newer to meditation may default to what they perceive as the "right" or logical response to inquiries, subtle messages about doing it "right," or missing the misperceptions about practice that often arise. This may result in missed opportunities for deeper understanding or experience among participants.

Also challenging for facilitators new to practice is the guiding of the meditation practices. Facilitators are strongly encouraged to guide from their own experience rather than reading the meditation instructions or attempting to induce a "meditative state." Facilitators with extensive experience with meditation practice are typically more at ease with guiding. This shifts the role of the facilitator from "teacher" to someone engaging in the practice alongside the participants, enhancing the collaborative feel and alliance of the groups. As stated by Kabat-Zinn (2003), "Without the foundation of personal practice and the embodying of what it is one is teaching, attempts at mindfulness-based interventions run the risk of becoming caricatures of mindfulness, missing the radical, transformational essence."

MBRP AND 12-STEP APPROACHES

Over the past decade, the ways in which MBRP can serve as either an alternative or as a complement to 12-step involvement have become increasingly evident. Twelve-step programs have long been the most accessible and common approach to addictions treatment, and their effects are immeasurable. For many, the labels, terms, and path to recovery outlined by a 12-step approach provide validation of their experiences, relief from confusion and shame, accountability, direction, and a strong sense of community. However, for others the same labels and processes may feel constraining, disempowering, or punitive or be misaligned with their beliefs and experiences. Some of the people who are drawn to MBRP are seeking an alternative. Others for whom 12-step has been a solid support have found MBRP serves as a useful supplement.

While there are distinct differences between these approaches, there are many areas of overlap in their underlying themes and structure, including an emphasis on acceptance, letting go of personal attempts to control things not under our control, importance of consistent connection to program practices, and the value of contemplative practice, such as prayer and meditation (see Griffin, 2004, for an in-depth discussion of these issues). The points on which they diverge center primarily on the foundational view of addiction. Alcoholics Anonymous (AA), Narcotics Anonymous (NA), and other 12-step approaches are based on a combination of the disease and spiritual models of addiction, which view substance abuse and dependence as chronic, progressive diseases of the brain (Spicer, 1993). Affected individuals are often encouraged to accept the label of "addict" or "alcoholic" and to admit powerlessness over this disease. They are encouraged to enlist the support of a higher power to aid them in their recovery. In contrast, the MBRP approach discourages the use of and identification with labels, positive or negative. It incorporates elements of cognitive-behavioral relapse prevention that focus on coping skills, exploring cognitive and behavioral antecedents of addictive behavior, and increasing self-efficacy (Marlatt & Donovan, 2005). These practices, taken together, are intended to foster a sense of agency and freedom, such that one's actions are arising from greater self-awareness, acceptance, and compassion.

Another difference between the 12-step model and MBRP lies in their approaches to abstinence. Commitment to abstinence goals is a requirement for participation in AA and NA, whereas in MBRP, although abstinence is often viewed as an ideal goal, it is not a requirement of treatment participation. Clients often set their individual goals, which may be total abstinence or may involve a more stepped approach toward abstinence or harm reduction.

In the cognitive-behavioral relapse prevention approach, relapse is expressly discussed, focusing on events preceding the initial use of a substance, or "lapse," as well as what happens following a lapse. According to this model, a lapse is often followed by what is referred to as the "abstinence violation effect," or the self-blame, guilt, and loss of control that is typically experienced after the violation of a self-imposed rule (e.g., an individual may have the thought "I have already failed, so I may as well go all the way"; Curry, Marlatt, & Gordon, 1987). This puts the individual at an increased risk of relapse. Relapse prevention emphasizes the seriousness of a lapse while encouraging individuals to recognize that they still have the choice to cope effectively following a lapse and to return to their initial goals (Marlatt & Witkiewitz, 2005).

Similarly, although MBRP strongly supports abstinence, it is up to participants to decide what, if any, changes they choose for themselves. Because MBRP is designed as an aftercare program, participants typically have already undergone treatment and thus may have clarified their own goals or have had to comply with the goals of a legal system or treatment program. The MBRP approach does not necessarily address "goals," however. The mindfulness-based practices encourage individuals to become familiar with their thoughts, emotional reactions, and behavioral patterns, and to see for themselves which are working in their lives and which are problematic or damaging. For some, this might result in reduction in or alteration of patterns of use, and for others it may result in complete abstinence. A lapse is seen as a common occurrence in the change process and represents a learning opportunity rather than a failure or a return to square one. The overarching focus of MBRP on increasing awareness, however, allows flexibility to consider the individual needs and objectives of varied treatment programs.

These differences may not be apparent for some people. For others, they might arise when discussing relapse. For example, in Session 6's discussion of the relapse cycle, a lapse, or single use, is differentiated from a return to a full-blown cycle of relapse. It is often useful at this point to turn the discussion over to the group rather than presenting a certain model or theory of relapse. Participants can share experiences of previous relapses and the specific events leading up to an initial lapse. This often initiates a more organic discussion of various points in the chain of events where there might have been opportunities to "pause," stepping out of the "automatic" mode and breaking the chain of habitual behavior. The approach is collaborative and tends to lead to a more natural and relevant discussion of the role of thoughts, as well as sensations and emotions, following an initial lapse, and the potential of mindfulness practices in changing this pattern.

Fundamentally, both the 12-step and MBRP approaches begin with a realization that one's present behavioral and cognitive habits are causing suffering, and that the "refuge" of substance use or other addictive behavior is ultimately a false one. Both programs encourage developing wisdom to discern what we can and cannot control and an acceptance of that which is not in our control. Finally, the programs similarly encourage recognition of factors that increase vulnerability to relapse or other problematic habitual behaviors, such as states of body and mind (e.g., lonely, tired). They appreciate the mind's tendency to attach to unhelpful patterns (e.g., "resentments" in the 12-step approach or judgments and stories in MBRP) that ultimately cause more suffering and increase risk of relapse.

LOGISTICS

In addition to the theoretical challenges that may arise, there are also practical challenges of conducting MBRP. In our experience, these have included scheduling, participant motivation, and barriers to daily mindfulness practice. We describe some issues that we and our colleagues have encountered, and a brief discussion of how we have navigated them.

Time

For those working within a treatment agency, there may be limitations to length and timing of groups. Two hours is usually sufficient to cover the material outlined for each session; however, a shorter duration limits either the practices or the discussions, whereas an additional 15 to 30 minutes allows for a more in-depth exploration of the experiences and observations that arise in group. When scheduling permits, we recommend longer sessions (2½-hour sessions are often used in MBSR and MBCT). Another common experience is difficulty scheduling an extended half- or full-day session during the course (see Part III on extended mindfulness practice). As any mindfulness practitioner who has been on intensive retreat knows, there are many merits to sustained periods of practice. However, constraints of scheduling and space for those working within treatment agencies or other institutional settings may not allow for this opportunity.

Legal and Motivational Issues

Over the years, we have worked with a variety of populations, including several who were either court mandated or "voluntold" to participate in an MBRP group. This has at times detracted from the honesty, openness, and nonjudgmental stance that MBRP is designed to cultivate and model. Additionally, it may prevent some participants from returning to the group following an instance of use. Ideally, groups include discussion of lapses that occur during the course of the treatment, allowing participants an experience of acceptance and support, even in the event of a lapse in abstinence. This provides an opportunity to observe the tendency of the mind in such a situation and to reinforce, as much as possible, letting go of judgment and beginning again.

There are a number of ways we have worked with this. When possible, we ask that no agency staff be present for the group, and that any information shared regarding use or relapse not be subject to punitive consequences. Another option is to speak hypothetically, or about patterns of use in the past, and be clear with the group about the intentions of this. Regarding motivation, we have found it most helpful to invite people in the very first session to be honest about why they are participating in the group. We encourage all responses and invite healthy skepticism.

Supporting Continuity through Daily Practice and Attendance

Full participation in group sessions and daily practice is essential to the integration of practice and related skills into daily life. Facilitation and support of daily mindfulness practice and regular group attendance are thus emphasized throughout the 8 weeks. Although using previously recorded meditations offered on our or other websites is an option for supporting daily practice, we encourage facilitators to create their own recordings. Participants often prefer to hear the familiar voices of their facilitators, and consistency between the in-session and recorded meditation instructions may support overall engagement with the practice. Additionally, participants may express a preference for a particular style or gender of voice to guide them through the meditation instructions. Finally, it can be useful to offer meditations of different lengths, or ones that use a vocabulary or style more appropriate for specific populations.

Participants' living situations may present additional barriers to daily practice. Some may be housed in challenging or unstable situations with consequent difficulties finding time and space for meditation practice, or they may not have access to playback equipment. In these instances, we have spent time in groups generating ideas for practice times and places. Although living conditions may remain a real barrier for some participants, many are able to work within the strictures of their situations and find creative ways to integrate formal practice into their daily lives, such as practicing on long bus rides or retreating to a library or a parked car, where they can take a break from the chaos of their environments to practice. Some agencies and clinics have designated on-site daily practice time and space to support participants' practice.

Regular attendance in groups is also essential to learning the mindfulness-based skills and practices. Not surprisingly, participants unable to attend sessions are often less engaged in subsequent sessions. We have found this especially true of attendance at the first two sessions; those who miss these initial sessions often have difficulty engaging as fully as other members. Despite attempts to "fill them in" on the material and practices covered in previous sessions, the shared experiences and group discussions are what offer a richer understanding of and engagement with the material.

Gender Composition and Group Size

The MBRP structured protocol does not specifically address group composition by gender; however, it is an issue worthy of consideration when organizing a group. Having facilitated both mixed-gender and gender-segregated groups, our experience indicates that some participants, particularly those with a history of interpersonal trauma, may benefit more from gender-specific groups.

In our experience, 8 to 12 participants is ideal, although we have facilitated groups of as few as 3 and as many as 18. A larger group size may result in decreased time for each individual to share experiences, questions, and concerns, and may present a challenge for facilitators in terms of completing all of the intended exercises while providing adequate time for inquiry. On the other hand, a small group (fewer than 6) means less opportunity for participants to learn from and be validated by others' experiences.

Precourse Meetings

In our efforts to increase retention and therapeutic alliance, coupled with the MBSR and MBCT practice of conducting initial interviews with prospective group members, we have found that holding brief individual meetings with each participant before the course begins can help assess and clarify expectations, providing rationale for the significant commitment the course requires and allowing an opportunity for prospective participants to raise questions or concerns.

We typically review the basic structure of the course (e.g., schedule, expectations, attendance), highlight the importance of home practice, and inquire about motivation and anticipated barriers to participation. It is helpful to elicit from individuals their own motivations and commitment rather than attempt to "sell" them on the course (which just doesn't work). Even these brief meetings seem to enhance interest and commitment, increase rapport, and improve attendance. For example, in one trial, participants who received a pretreatment brief motivational interview, compared to those who didn't, were significantly more likely to show up for the first MBRP session (Grow, 2013).

ADDITIONAL ISSUES TO CONSIDER

Although we have learned substantial and invaluable lessons throughout the process of designing, training, implementing, and evaluating MBRP, there are many areas and issues that we continue to explore, several of which we discuss below.

Lovingkindness

Metta, or lovingkindness, is a core practice in the Theravada tradition, where vipassana meditation has its roots. The practice typically involves bringing attention to a set of phrases intended to cultivate friendliness and kindness toward oneself, friends, and loved ones; strangers or "neutral" people; those who are challenging; and finally toward all beings.

Self-judgment and self-criticism are pervasive and palpable in our culture, and perhaps even more so among individuals with histories of addictive behavior. Not only do these individuals often internalize the judgment and stigma they have experienced from society and family, but they frequently have great difficulty forgiving themselves for the negative consequences that have arisen as a result of their substance use or other behaviors. Thus, we appreciate the need for cultivation of friendliness and warmth toward oneself as central to recovery and healing. We include aspects of metta and forgiveness in several of the meditation instructions, and a formal metta practice in the final two sessions. In the MBRP program, we often refer to this practice as "kindness," rather than metta or "lovingkindness," depending on the population and how we anticipate such terms might be received. Some may have resistance or expectations associated with the word "love," which is typically associated with romantic love. We also modify the domains (i.e., do not include the neutral or difficult person) and just practice sending well-wishes to a loved one, followed by sending those to oneself. The focus is on noticing one's experiences while doing this, rather than an attempt to cultivate a particular emotion or feeling.

Posture in Practices

Posture during practices, which might seem a minor issue, can be helpful to address. Although some participants may choose to sit in chairs because of physical concerns, many may choose to use cushions or mats on the floor. A facilitator joining those on the floor often creates an atmosphere of familiarity and shared experience, shifting the role of the facilitators from authorities to fellow meditation practitioners. However, it may also inadvertently foster the notion that mindfulness practice requires adopting a special posture, is outside of an individual's cultural context or framework, or is something that is primarily practiced "on the cushion" rather than in daily life. Sitting or lying down on the floor may also increase drowsiness or laxity in posture. Having a single zafu or similar cushion for each participant, placed underneath each chair, may allow experimentation with sitting postures while also maintaining some of the formality of practice. However, in the event that cushions are unavailable, all of the practices can be engaged in while seated in a chair. We recommend that facilitators experiment in their groups and find what feels best suited to themselves and their participants. We also recommend, especially in early sessions, sharing the intention of posture (i.e., using the body to help cultivate certain attitudes or qualities of attention in the mind).

Common Misconceptions

The increased popularity of mindfulness practice in the broader culture over the past decade has resulted in a proliferation of the language and some of the practices in popular culture. This has many potential benefits, and also some potential causes for concern. The popularization has included messaging around what practice should look like, and who has access to practice and who doesn't. How many photos have we seen on magazine covers of thin, conventionally attractive young women in flowing white clothing sitting on a mountain or beach in a perfect seated pose, with a blissful smile on their face? These depictions foster unfortunate misunderstandings and expectations about mindfulness practice that often accompany participants as they walk into Session 1. We find it useful to name these common misconceptions up front. For example, mindfulness practice does not mean always having a calm and quiet mind, experiencing bliss, having to sit in a certain posture, only practicing under certain conditions, and so forth. As facilitators, we also keep eyes and ears open for when these misconceptions arise throughout the course, often in the process of inquiry. Sometimes they are directly expressed ("That practice didn't work for me, I couldn't feel calm") and other times show up in more veiled ways, such as doubt about oneself or the practice, being disengaged, or lack of attendance. These doubts and expectations, like anything else, can be turned into objects of awareness. Participants often worry (though they may not say it out loud without encouragement from the facilitator) that their mind is uniquely unsuited for mindfulness practice because it wanders or gets distracted. Naming the misconceptions and validating the participants' awareness helps normalize their experiences.

Working with Trauma

The significant increase in research on mindfulness-based interventions since the first edition of this book has brought with it been a great deal more awareness of and attention to the potential risks or "side effects" of mindfulness practice for people with trauma histories. This is one of the most common questions we are asked at our trainings or conference presentations. Given the high rates of trauma in the general population, as well as the high co-occurrence of trauma-related symptoms in populations with substance use disorder, it is probably safe to assume that many participants in MBRP groups have trauma histories that they may have previously self-medicated with substances. Although creating a safe environment is imperative for all participants, it is critical for those with trauma histories or for whom safety and trust are significant concerns. Above all, the intentions of the practices need to be kept at the forefront: to cultivate curiosity, clear seeing, and compassion. We are observing our experiences—particularly those that are painful—with curiosity, presence, and gentleness, so as to practice a different way of relating to them. Although often uncomfortable and challenging, these practices should never feel threatening and are thus best fostered in a safe, supported context. Here are some specific ways to create such a context:

Permission and Choice

It is vital to offer participants choices in how they practice or engage with their experience by providing options and using language that suggests an invitation rather than a command or directive, which may be experienced as authoritative, disrespectful, or disempowering. For example, the facilitator might say: "You may choose to keep your eyes open or closed for this practice. If you choose to close your eyes, know that you may open them at any point if this feels more comfortable for you. You are also welcome to adopt any posture that is supportive and comfortable for you, including sitting or standing up." We also need to recognize that sensations of breathing may not be a neutral anchor for some people, and that other anchors, such as the soles of the feet on the ground or the sensations in the hands, are equally suitable options.

Zones of Engagement

Although many MBRP practices involve approaching experiences of discomfort, it is equally important, and perhaps even more so for those with trauma histories, to learn to bring awareness to internal cues to "step back" when something is overwhelming or no longer allows for kindness or stability of attention. Learning this may require some practice and may need repeated encouragement. It can also be an important vehicle for healing, especially for those who have had experiences of feeling unsafe in their bodies, having boundaries violated, and experiencing general disempowerment or lack of agency.

Relatedly, it is helpful in the first session or two, and especially in the context of the Urge Surfing exercise, to discuss the "three zones" of engagement. These include the Habit/Comfort zone, where we avoid thoughts, feelings, and sensations that are challenging, but where there is also little to no growth; the Challenge zone, where we may experience discomfort, but it is workable and there is the potential for change and growth; and the zone where we are in a state of Overwhelm (see Figure I.2). This last state is not productive and may actually cause damage. These zones are similar to the spectrum of physical exercise and health, where sitting on the couch may be comfortable and feel safe but does not improve strength or flexibility. If we push ourselves too hard, however, we might risk tearing a muscle or harming our bodies in some way. There is a middle zone, where we can gently challenge the limits of comfort in a way that improves our strength and flexibility. This is where optimal growth and strength building occur.

Several of the practices and exercises in MBRP invite us out of our Habit/Comfort zone into the Challenge zone and thus may involve some uncomfortable feelings and sensations. This shift in our relationship to discomfort and stretching of our capacity to "be with," instead of immediately reacting or attempting to "fix," is at the heart of MBRP. However, this is not the same as diving into the deep end or having forced contact with something that is overwhelming or harmful. Challenge must be balanced with skillful kindness. This might include taking an intentional step back from potential overwhelm by opening the eyes, focusing attention on the feet, hands, or the breath, bringing awareness to sights and sounds in the room, and/or moving around. We frequently remind participants that these techniques are available to them.

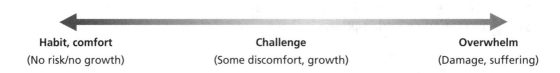

Habit, comfort	Challenge	Overwhelm
(No risk/no growth)	(Some discomfort, growth)	(Damage, suffering)

FIGURE I.2. Zones of engagement.

Modified Practices

The practices in this book (both structure and wording) are based on our experiences with participants with whom we have worked. However, as this program becomes more widely used, we recognize and support the need to modify structure, form, language, and style to best suit the individuals engaging in them. If we as facilitators understand the intentions of the practices, we also understand that the way in which they are presented can be flexible. There are many ways to practice placing attention onto physical sensations in the body, for example, or to practice observing thoughts in the mind rather than getting caught up in them. For example, as discussed above, for participants with trauma histories, closing one's eyes or lying down may be overwhelming or threatening. Practicing sitting in a chair or even standing (especially with practices like the body scan) and keeping eyes open during practices should be offered as options. When we are working with youth, who often have difficulty with the longer practices in which instructions are often about stillness and bringing awareness to more subtle experiences, practices might involve more movement and playfulness, or be broken up into shorter segments of instructions. We might offer movement or walking instead of sitting or body scans for home practice.

PART II

Facilitator's Guide

As described in Part I, this program is designed to be facilitated by clinicians with an established foundation in mindfulness meditation, an ongoing daily practice, and, ideally, formal training in MBRP, MBSR, or MBCT. We strongly suggest that readers begin with Part I before continuing on to the treatment guide to better understand the history and intentions of the program.

The following chapters offer a framework for those wishing to facilitate MBRP groups. Although we have included example scripts for meditation practices, these are intended only as suggestions to help facilitators get a better feel for guidance. Before each script, we list the primary intentions of that particular practice. As mentioned in the Introduction, a facilitator's engagement and presence in leading each of these practices is an opportunity to model the embodiment of the qualities of spontaneity, presence, and openness to one's own arising experiences. This offers authenticity that can be lost when reading from a script, and can exemplify the "trust in experience" and present-centeredness that are foundational to MBRP. We thus encourage facilitators to participate in all meditation exercises while leading them, guiding from their own experience rather than simply giving instructions or reading from a book.

OVERVIEW OF SESSIONS

The following chapters outline each of the eight sessions (see Table II.1). Chapters include an overview of the topics and themes included in each session, a detailed discussion of the practices and exercises, and a description of the experiences and challenges that often arise. We include excerpted dialogue to clarify and aid in the illustration of themes, practices, and discussions. The specific exercises and

TABLE II.1. Sessions in the MBRP Program

Session 1: Automatic Pilot and Mindful Awareness

Session 2: A New Relationship with Discomfort

Session 3: From Reacting to Responding

Session 4: Mindfulness in Challenging Situations

Session 5: Acceptance and Skillful Action

Session 6: Seeing Thoughts as Thoughts

Session 7: Supporting and Sustaining Well-Being

Session 8: Social Support and Continuing Practice

handouts listed and discussed in each session are included at the end of each chapter.

Although each session has a central theme, each is intended to build upon the previous weeks' materials and practices. The course begins with an experiential introduction to the tendency toward "automatic pilot." Exercises and discussions in the first three sessions center on this theme. By bringing awareness to this deeply habitual tendency, and through specific practices designed to bring attention to the present, participants begin recognizing and stepping out of this automatic mode, both in session and in their daily lives. Awareness of the role of automatic pilot in relapse is also discussed in these initial sessions. Sessions 4 to 6 explore the application of practices learned thus far to situations in which participants might be at increased risk of relapse or reactive behavior. These sessions identify individual risk profiles and involve integrating mindfulness skills into these situations. Finally, Sessions 7 and 8 widen the lens, looking at the bigger picture of creating and maintaining a lifestyle that will support both recovery and mindfulness practice.

The first formal practice introduced in the course is the body scan exercise. Throughout the 8 weeks, this focus on the body remains central and is revisited through practices such as walking meditation, mindful movement, and inquiry. The body is the first foundation of mindfulness, providing a reliable way of bringing attention into the present moment. This practice also presents an opportunity to observe how the mind responds to uncomfortable experiences, learning how to "be with" discomfort and craving rather than reacting in habitual avoidant and often destructive ways. The practices gradually progress to working with emotional discomfort, encouraging greater gentleness and acceptance of one's internal experience. Once participants have had some experience observing sensations and emotional states, they are introduced to the observation of thoughts as objects of awareness. In the final sessions, practices centered on the active cultivation of kindness and compassion are introduced.

BEGINNING AND ENDING EACH SESSION

Before the start of each session, facilitators will naturally be planning the specific structure and preparing materials for the session. In addition, we've found that when we as facilitators engage in even a brief period of personal meditation just prior to the session, we have increased ease, awareness, and presence in the group and enter the room in a calmer, clearer state of mind.

Sessions can easily end with a flurry of papers, scheduling details, and rushed gathering of belongings. Continuation of practice into daily life can be further supported by inviting participants at the close of each session to stop wherever they are, without the need to shift into any special posture, and take a brief pause to focus on the breath, on sounds, or on what is happening in their bodies. They can then be encouraged to stay with this awareness as they gather their things and move into the rest of their day or evening.

Automatic Pilot and Mindful Awareness

Stepping out of the busyness, stopping our endless pursuit of
getting somewhere else, is perhaps the most beautiful offering
we can make to our spirit.

—Tara Brach

Materials

- Bell
- Whiteboard/markers
- Raisins, bowl, spoon
- Handout 1.1: Overview of Sessions
- Handout 1.2: Session 1 Theme and Daily Practice: Automatic Pilot and Mindful Awareness
- Handout 1.3: Daily Practice Tracking Sheet
- Audio File: Body Scan

Theme

When we experience cravings and urges, we often engage in reactive or impulsive behaviors, without full awareness of what is occurring and what the consequences might be. This first session introduces the idea of "automatic pilot," or acting without awareness, and explores the relationships among automatic pilot, mindful awareness, and relapse. We begin with a practice to help recognize this tendency and learn how to begin shifting from habitual and often self-defeating behavior to observation of what is happening in our minds and bodies without "automatically" reacting. This session uses the "raisin exercise" to introduce mindful awareness using the senses, and contrast this with automatic pilot. Body scan practice is then introduced as a way of bringing attention to present-moment experiences in the body.

Goals

- Establish guidelines for participation in the group.
- Discuss structure of the group.
- Explore mindful awareness versus "automatic pilot."
- Introduce the body scan as a way of bringing awareness to physical experience.

Session Outline

- Introductions
- Expectations and Agreements for the Group
- Group Structure and Format
- Raisin Exercise (Practice 1.1): Automatic Pilot and Mindful Awareness
- What Is Mindfulness?
- Body Scan Meditation (Practice 1.2)
- Daily Practice
- Closing

Practice for This Week

- Body scan
- Mindfulness of daily activities
- Daily Practice Tracking Sheet

The primary intention of this first session is to introduce some basics of mindfulness practice, to offer an experiential sense of the automatic pilot mode, and to begin discriminating between automatic versus mindful awareness. The session also introduces the relationship between automatic or reactive behavior and relapse. Participants explore basic components of mindful awareness through practices that encourage slowing down, bringing attention to present-moment experience, and observing the mind and the different senses.

INTRODUCTIONS

In this first session, facilitators set the tone for the group and create a space that supports exploration and presence. To emphasize the experiential nature of the course, it is helpful to keep beginning logistics and explanations brief. Introductions, too, are typically limited to name and (briefly) reason for participating in the course. Facilitators may initiate introductions by having participants take a moment to reflect on what is important to them at this juncture in their lives, asking, "What do you most value about being here? If this course could help you have the life you wanted, what would shift?"

EXPECTATIONS FOR GROUP AND GROUP AGREEMENTS

Rather than dictating rules to the group, we ask participants what factors will help ensure a sense of safety and comfort and facilitate participation and engagement in the course. Components that often arise are consistency in attendance, notifying facilitators in advance of any absences, confidentiality, commitment to the work and the process, honesty, a nonjudgmental attitude, and other issues involving basic respect for other group members' needs and experiences. In addition, we have found it helpful to discuss the value of speaking from one's own experience rather than making assumptions about the experience of others, recognizing that people in the group may be at different stages in the change process, and inviting people to bring awareness to their tendencies in a group context (e.g., speaking more or faster when anxious, or pulling back). These agreements are then listed on the board and lay the groundwork for participation. Having this conversation up front strengthens group cohesion and fosters an attitude of respect, commitment, and engagement in making the group most conducive to full participation. We have found it helpful to save this list and refer back to these agreements at the start of future sessions, if and as needed.

GROUP STRUCTURE AND FORMAT

Basic structure and logistics of the course, such as schedule and breaks, are important to review, and also best kept brief so the experiential nature of the program is emphasized in this beginning session. We let participants know that the group may differ from other groups they've experienced, as discussions tend to focus on present experiences rather than stories about the past week, ideas, conceptual thinking, or "processing." We also ask permission in this first session to pause and redirect if we notice someone is relaying a story or talking about events, versus talking about their direct experience. We clarify that this isn't because we don't want to know about people's lives, but because we are most interested in how events are experienced, that is, the sensations, thoughts, and emotions that arise in these circumstances. Stepping in and redirecting is a way to begin shifting focus from external details of an event to our own internal experiences and reactions. We have found this to be a helpful way for participants to give permission for us to pause and redirect, and they understand that it is not an interruption so much as an expression of curiosity about their experiences. Facilitators also explain that sessions are rich in material and exercises, and that each person may not have the opportunity to share his or her experience following every exercise. Given that similar themes and exercises are covered repeatedly (Handout 1.1), all participants will have a chance at some point to share experiences.

It is suggested that, as best they can, participants suspend judgments or ideas about the value of these practices until the end of the course, bringing a willingness to experience whatever arises with curiosity and openness. At the end of the 8 weeks, they will have the opportunity to assess the value of these practices in their lives and can choose whether or not to continue. As long as they are committed to attending the course, they are asked to "jump in" and participate fully.

In beginning discussions of daily practice, it is useful for participants to understand that the in-session practices are only an introduction and that, although they will inevitably learn from these alone, this course is most powerful when these practices are integrated into their daily lives, which takes some commitment and effort, especially in the beginning. It is also helpful in this conversation to highlight the importance of attendance. Each session builds on themes and exercises from previous weeks; thus, attending group each week and engaging in the daily practices between sessions are crucial to the program. Another topic to discuss is the use of substances during the course of the program. We recognize that people are at different stages of change, and participants are strongly encouraged to return to the group following a slip or a relapse (provided this doesn't necessitate return to a higher level of care). However, they are asked to refrain from attending the group while under the influence of a substance.

RAISIN EXERCISE/AUTOMATIC PILOT
AND MINDFUL AWARENESS

Each session begins with a mindfulness practice, followed by inquiry-style discussion in which experiences and themes are elicited from participants. Discussions are guided using primarily open-ended questions and facilitated from a nonjudgmental, present-centered stance that is reflective of the practice itself.

Similar to the MBSR and MBCT programs, the first experiential exercise in

MBRP involves mindfully observing and eating a single raisin (Practice 1.1).* The raisin exercise is an opportunity to mindfully engage in an activity that many people have performed countless times, often without much awareness. Slowing down and bringing an intentional, curious attention to the sensations, thoughts, urges, and even emotions involved in this simple activity illustrates how a typically automatic behavior, when observed, can offer a rich array of sensory experiences, as well as reactions of either "liking/wanting" or "disliking/aversion." It allows participants to experience the difference between mindful attention and a more habitual automatic mode and provides an opportunity to explore the relationships between automatic pilot, addiction, and relapse.

Following the exercise, facilitators inquire about participants' experiences, including sensations, thoughts, feelings, and urges, as well as any reactions to those experiences, such as judgment, aversion, or pleasure. The primary focus is on the direct experience, with facilitators redirecting where necessary. Participants reliably comment on how they have never "really tasted" a raisin or observed the nuances of it, or how they typically eat a handful without even being aware that they have consumed them. This sometimes progresses to discussion of the parallels between this experience and blindly following a craving or an urge without attention to the numerous steps and reactions involved in the downward spiral.

This is illustrated in the following example:

FACILITATOR: What did people notice in doing this exercise?

PARTICIPANT 1: I started thinking about how this raisin was alive at one time, and noticing it had seeds in it. My mind automatically went to "grape—this was a grape. Now it's a raisin."

FACILITATOR: So thoughts arose about the history of this object. It seems like you noticed some of the more subtle things about the object as well, like the seeds.

PARTICIPANT 2: I noticed the color, a beautiful red. It looked like one side was shriveled with tiny, tiny seeds and the other side was shiny. Then my mind went off to pretending I was beaming information back to another planet. Then my mind came back. I was excited when you said, "Put it in your mouth."

FACILITATOR: You noticed a lot of different things. The color and texture of the object, the tendency of the mind to wander off into a fantasy or thought. Also seems like you were aware of that, and were able to bring

---

*In some of our groups, we have substituted a dried cranberry because raisins may have associations with wine for some of our participants. Although this association may offer a rich opportunity for paying attention to the experience of craving, we intend to keep this first introduction simple. Mindful observation of craving is addressed later in the program.

your attention back to the moment. And then you said you were excited when you got to eat the raisin.

PARTICIPANT 2: Yes, but once I bit into it, though, I didn't like the way it tasted.

FACILITATOR: When you say you didn't like how it tasted, what happened? How did you experience "not liking"?

PARTICIPANT 2: When it got to the back of my throat before I swallowed, there was a reaction in my mouth, my throat and mouth, that was not a pleasant taste, and I thought "I don't like it."

FACILITATOR: So both a physical reaction and the thought "I don't like this"?

PARTICIPANT 3: I had the thought that I wanted some more.

FACILITATOR: Ahh, okay. So an awareness that this experience would end, and a desire for it to continue, to have more. Is that a familiar experience for you?

PARTICIPANT 3: (*Laughs*) Yes, it sure is.

In this discussion, the facilitator highlights the direct sensory experiences, gently redirecting comments that wander into stories or reactions. The facilitator also distinguishes between thoughts and sensations. The intention is for participants not only to bring their awareness to present-moment experience but also to become aware of the tendency of the mind to wander away from the moment and to learn to gently guide it back without judgment. Further, the idea of thoughts being "objects of awareness" rather than facts or truths is introduced. The facilitator also inquires whether the participant's experience (a desire for something to continue) is a familiar one.

FACILITATOR: So let me ask: All these details, is this something you would typically notice when eating a raisin?

PARTICIPANT 1: No, I never have before. I'd just eat it.

FACILITATOR: How is this different than how you normally eat a raisin?

PARTICIPANT 1: I just shove a bunch in my mouth.

FACILITATOR: So speed is part of it; you usually eat faster.

PARTICIPANT 1: Yeah, especially when I come home at night I just eat, and I'm not usually paying attention.

FACILITATOR: So your mind is maybe elsewhere, not on what you are actually doing?

PARTICIPANT 1: Right. I already know what I'm eating so I don't pay attention, I don't look at it. I've done this a thousand times.

PARTICIPANT 2: Yeah, I've never slowed down like that, looked at it, felt it, appreciated it.

PARTICIPANT 1: It's kind of like when you've been locked up [incarcerated] and you finally get your freedom back. When you have it, you don't appreciate it. But when it's taken away, you understand freedom again, you suddenly appreciate everything, you notice everything you used to just take for granted.

FACILITATOR: All these things you used to take for granted you suddenly notice and appreciate—even these so-called "little" things. There may be some connection between that and freedom for you—interesting.

So you mentioned this idea of it being "automatic"—you've done it a thousand times before, not paying attention. Every week's session has a theme, and this week's theme is exactly what you're bringing up here: "automatic pilot." Can you think of other examples of times in your life when you're on automatic pilot?

PARTICIPANT 3: Driving to work—it's like, "What happened back there?" That whole time disappeared.

The prior dialogue again illustrates the facilitator's intention to elicit ideas and themes from participants rather than "teaching" them or attempting to stress the importance of the practice or all the great things about mindfulness. By asking how the experience with the raisin contrasts with their typical way of doing things, the facilitator encourages participants to become more aware of their tendency to live on automatic pilot. In our experience, these key themes reliably arise from discussion with some gentle direction, open questions, and a focus on present-moment experience. This gradually moves to the distinction between this and typical experience and, finally, the relationship of this experience to relapse. We have also found it helpful to draw all participants into the group, often highlighting the "nonpersonal" nature of an individual's experience by asking whether others in the group experienced something similar or different. Typically, experiences are shared by several group members. Finally, the facilitator brings the exercise into the context of relapse, again by eliciting from the group rather than teaching:

FACILITATOR: So why do you think are we doing this exercise in a relapse-prevention group? Does this have anything at all to do with relapse or addiction?

PARTICIPANT 1: When I start drinking, I'm already on automatic pilot. It's something I've done a million times. I already know where I'm going to go, what I'm going to do. It's not conscious.

PARTICIPANT 2: For me it happens way before I actually use [drugs]. It might be a month previous, a little thought pops into my mind or I do something . . . like I used to sell drugs but not use them. But in the scheme of things I knew I was going to use eventually. It was a huge lie to myself. If you don't stop and pay attention, you can be on that road without even seeing it.

FACILITATOR: So slowing down and noticing where we are and what our minds are doing—bringing some awareness to what is happening in the moment might help us make more skillful choices.

Throughout this course, we will practice awareness of sensations, thoughts, and emotions, specifically in relation to cravings and relapse. We will practice new ways to relate to these experiences, especially difficult ones, so that we don't just default to our habitual ways. We are not trying to get rid of all difficult experiences, because that's not possible; we are learning to relate to them differently so we have more choice in how we respond. So maybe they don't have as much control over us.

WHAT IS MINDFULNESS?

Following the exercise, we ask participants to describe mindfulness, based on what they have just experienced. Participants often point to qualities of awareness, choice, present-centered focus or "being in the moment," ability to stop habitual responses, and feelings of connection. We recommend writing these on a whiteboard, noting themes that emerge. Based on their descriptions, we come up with a working definition of mindfulness that contains the core components: intentional cultivation of attention aimed at present-moment experience, with an attitude of gentleness, curiosity, and kindness. This can be a good place to discuss the common misconceptions of mindfulness practice (e.g., feeling bliss, having no thoughts; see the "Common Misconceptions" section in Part I).

The aspects of paying attention and focusing on present-moment experience have often been offered by participants in the discussion. The quality of gentleness and kindness toward one's experience, however, frequently goes unmentioned. We might highlight this aspect of the practice repeatedly throughout the course: Mindful attention is not only about paying attention to what is occurring but also about having compassion and, as best we can, adopting a nonjudgmental stance toward whatever is arising. For example, when aversive reactions to the raisin exercise arise, it can be an excellent first opportunity to highlight awareness of aversion and to model a curious and nonjudgmental stance even toward that which we don't like.

BODY SCAN MEDITATION

Similar to the MBSR and MBCT programs, the first formal meditation practice in the course is the body scan meditation (Practice 1.2). In the vipassana, or insight meditative tradition from which many of the MBRP practices originate, awareness of the body is described as the first foundation of mindfulness. In many of the MBRP practices, we return to sensations in the body as a way of stepping out of the stories in which we have become entangled and returning to the present moment. As with the raisin exercise, we emphasize openness to and curiosity about any and all experiences that arise during the body scan practice, disabusing ourselves of expectations about what one should or shouldn't experience and reminding participants that the intention is to pay attention to experience, whatever it may be, and to repeatedly return attention to the body each time it wanders (which it will).

In the context of relapse prevention, the practice of paying attention to physical experience can be especially valuable, because experiences of reactivity, cravings, and urges often manifest physically before the subsequent chain of thoughts or reactions. When in automatic pilot mode, we often lose contact with the immediate physical experience. Thus, coming back to physical sensations is a way of reconnecting with present experience and can be a first step in shifting from habitual, reactive behavior to making more mindful and skillful choices.

Because this is the first "formal" practice in which participants engage, we offer a number of choices of posture, including sitting in a chair with eyes either open or closed. While lying down may be presented as an option, this may be too vulnerable a position or feel unsafe for a number of people, particularly those with a history of trauma (see the "Working with Trauma" section in Part I). Further, it may be helpful to give participants permission to stand if they choose to, open their eyes at any time, or shift positions.

Rather than doing one longer body scan practice, we have sometimes found it helpful to start with a brief body scan (e.g., just bringing awareness to the soles of the feet for a few minutes) and then a brief period of inquiry. This can then be followed by a longer body scan practice. For many participants, this will be their first formal practice, and a brief introductory practice and inquiry allow the facilitator to identify and address misconceptions (e.g., "my mind was all over the place, so something must be wrong") or answer questions before engaging in the longer body scan. It can also help participants' confidence in their ability to "meditate."

The template offered is an example rather than a script and can be adjusted to best suit your group, adhering to the intention of the body scan, rather than to the specific form or phrases.

In the inquiry following the body scan, participants typically express a range of responses, from peace and relaxation to restlessness and physical discomfort. The following is an example of inquiry following this practice:

FACILITATOR: What were people's observations and experiences?

PARTICIPANT 1: That was really relaxing.

FACILITATOR: What did you notice in your body or mind that was "relaxing"?

PARTICIPANT 1: Just like a sensation of release and breathing more deeply.

FACILITATOR: Okay, thank you. What else did people notice?

PARTICIPANT 2: I noticed that early on my mind was wandering away from the area we were focusing on, but later on it wasn't drifting as much.

FACILITATOR: Ah, yes. Did anyone else notice the mind wandering off to other things?

In this example, the facilitator begins with the first level of inquiry by focusing on the experience of "relaxing." She then addresses the nonpersonal nature of a participant's response to normalize or validate an experience (mind wandering) that could easily elicit self-judgment and to counter the possible assumption that something "went wrong." She offers recognition of this tendency of the mind ("Ah, yes"), followed by inquiring whether this experience was shared ("Did anyone else notice the mind wandering?"). A facilitator may even offer his or her own experience with the practice to reduce misconceptions or illustrate the universality of this tendency. Finally, as the discussion continues, she inquires about reactions or judgments to the experience of mind wandering. As illustrated, all levels of inquiry are not necessarily touched upon in every interaction and are not necessarily in a set order:

FACILITATOR: For those of you who noticed the mind wandering, what happened when you noticed that? Was there a reaction?

PARTICIPANT 1: Well, when I found myself off somewhere else, I realized I wasn't doing what I was supposed to be doing.

FACILITATOR: So you were aware of your mind wandering, and then had a thought like "I'm not doing what I'm supposed to be doing"?

PARTICIPANT 2: Yeah, like, "I'm doing this wrong."

FACILITATOR: Okay, thank you. Anyone else notice any self-judgment?

PARTICIPANT 2: Yeah, I noticed some too.

FACILITATOR: The instruction here is to notice that "I'm doing this wrong" is a thought, and gently bring your attention back to the body. As we discussed earlier, mindfulness is not about *not having* thoughts or the mind *not* wandering, but about being aware of *whatever* is happening. So if the mind wanders a hundred times, we simply notice that and return to the body here in the present moment a hundred times.

There are often experiences of drowsiness and sleepiness that arise:

PARTICIPANT: I was struggling to stay awake because I was so relaxed.

FACILITATOR: Ah yes, anyone else feel sleepy? What did that sleepiness or struggle to stay awake feel like for you?

PARTICIPANT: I found that I would sort of drift off and then have a moment of being startled and waking up again.

FACILITATOR: Were there thoughts that you noticed in that moment of waking up?

PARTICIPANT: I thought "Oh no—I need to stay awake."

FACILITATOR: So some judgment? When we lie down and close our eyes, it's often a signal for our bodies and minds to fall asleep, especially if we are tired. We can bring curiosity to the experience of sleepiness. "What does sleepiness feel like? What is it like to drift into and come out of sleep? What thoughts are arising about the experience?" If sleepiness arises repeatedly, it might be helpful to do the practice sitting up in a more alert posture, or to open the eyes a little to let some light in—these may be things to experiment with this week.

Again, the facilitator validates the experience and provides insights and strategies based on her or his own experience while remaining curious and nonjudgmental. The balance here is delicate, offering some skillful ways of working with challenges while still keeping the focus on present-moment experience rather than "doing it right" or "fixing" it.

DAILY PRACTICE

The first session establishes the tone for the remainder of the course by emphasizing integration of the practices from each session into daily life (Handout 1.2), while continuing to foster the nonjudgmental environment of the group. The importance of practice can be illustrated with analogies such as working daily to build a muscle, which gradually builds strength, or asking for an example of a skill at which a participant is adept and inquiring how he or she acquired that skill. We emphasize that the amount of benefit derived is related to participants' commitment to practicing. They are encouraged to commit to the course fully for these 8 weeks, and a core part of this is the daily practice. This is balanced, however, with a clear message that they will not be judged or evaluated on their practice. The Daily Practice Tracking Sheet (Handout 1.3) is presented as a way for participants to attend to what they are learning from the course and to note experiences that arise in the process rather than as an evaluative measure. These tracking sheets also allow facilitators to learn more about what is happening over the week and respond to any concerns or barriers that arose.

MINDFULNESS OF DAILY ACTIVITY

Again, in the tradition of MBSR and MBCT, one of the suggested daily practices for this first week is to bring the same qualities of attention, awareness, and curiosity as were brought to eating the raisin to a routine activity, such as brushing teeth or washing dishes. As with the raisin exercise, the suggestion is to bring attention to the activity as though experiencing it for the first time, using all of the senses. We have typically provided participants with a few examples and then asked them to generate their own, either picking the same activity to repeat each day or choosing different activities throughout the week. This is simply a way for participants to begin integrating mindfulness into their lives, incorporating moments of awareness throughout their days.

Occasionally, a participant will ask about "mindfully" using alcohol or drugs. We often respond by addressing the typically habitual and reactive aspects of substance use. Although it is true that we can bring close attention and awareness to any experience, including substance use, as practice deepens, awareness often develops of all the steps that occur before using, such as the cravings, thoughts, and feelings of discomfort that often trigger substance use. We might become aware of emotions that drive these cravings, such as fear, boredom, or loneliness, and have compassion for our own suffering and a willingness to feel it, rather than a reactive need to fix or escape it that leads to undesired consequences. This clear seeing allows us to make more skillful choices, noticing ways we increase our suffering and learning ways to reduce it.

CLOSING

To encourage continuity of awareness, we end each session with a few moments of silence followed by the bell. The facilitator might offer very brief guidance, such as awareness of body or breath, or just have the group sit in silence for a few moments and notice their experience, depending on the needs and feel of the group.

Raisin Exercise
PRACTICE 1.1

Intentions

+ Introduce mindfulness by bringing all senses to an external, tangible object
+ Experientially discern between "automatic pilot" and mindful awareness
+ Explore the relationship between automatic/reactive behavior and substance use/relapse

I'm going to pass some objects around. Go ahead and take two or three and just hold them in the palm of your hand. This is an exercise in noticing our experience, as best we can. So even as I pass these around, you might notice what is happening for you already—any thoughts you are having about what is happening? Any feelings of curiosity? Resistance? Do you notice anything happening in your body?

Now, I invite you to choose one of these objects and, as best you can, bring your full attention to this one object for the next few minutes. First, you might just notice which object you picked. Was there something about this one in particular that drew your attention? Maybe it was the biggest? The prettiest? Or maybe you chose one you felt sorry for. Or maybe you just picked one automatically.

Now look at this object carefully as though you have never seen anything like it. Bringing your attention to seeing it, maybe picking it up with the other hand and observing all its qualities, the way kids sometimes examine new things with innocent and focused curiosity.

You might feel its texture between your fingers, noticing its color and surfaces, and its unique shape.

While you are doing this, you might be aware, too, of thoughts you are having about this object, or about the exercise, or about how you are doing in the exercise. You might notice feelings like pleasure or maybe dislike for this object or this exercise. Noticing these thoughts or feelings as well and, as best you can, bringing your attention back to simply exploring this object.

You might bring this object up under your nose and inhale, noticing if it has a smell. You could even bring it to your ear and squish it a little and see if it has a sound. And now taking another look at it.

And now slowly bringing this object up to your mouth, aware of the arm moving the hand to position it correctly. And then gently placing the object against your lower lip, sensing how it feels there. Holding it there for a moment, aware of the sensations and any reactions. Maybe there's anticipation, or the mouth might be beginning to salivate.

Now placing this object on your tongue, and pausing here to feel what this object feels like in the mouth. The surfaces, texture, even the temperature of this object. Now beginning with just one bite into this object and pausing again there. Noticing what tastes are released, if the texture has changed. Maybe the object has now become two objects.

Now chewing slowly, noting the actual taste and change in texture. Maybe noticing, too, how the tongue and jaw work together to position the object between the teeth, how the tongue knows exactly where to position it as you chew.

And when you feel ready to swallow, watching that impulse to swallow. Pausing here before swallowing to notice the urge. What does that feel like? Are there thoughts?

Then, as you swallow the object, as best you can, feeling it as it travels down the throat and into the belly.

What is happening now? Maybe there is a leftover taste on the tongue. Maybe there is a relief that it is over, or perhaps a craving for more of these objects.

Based on Kabat-Zinn (1990).

Body Scan Meditation
PRACTICE 1.2

Intentions

✦ Awareness of body sensations as a way to connect with present-moment experience

✦ Openness and curiosity toward all experiences, versus expectations about what "should" or "shouldn't" be happening

✦ Exploring relevance of bringing attention to physical experience and reactivity, cravings, and urges

✦ Shifting the focus of attentional training from an outside object (raisin) to the interoceptive experience of the body, and intentionally moving awareness from one area of focus to another

---

You may choose to have your eyes open or closed for this practice. If you choose to have them open, find a spot in front of you, on the floor if you are sitting (or perhaps on the ceiling of you are lying down), so you are not looking around, but just allowing your gaze to rest.

We are going to explore the sensations through the whole body. As I guide you through, starting with the feet and moving all the way up to the head, the intention is to just notice what sensations are there. The idea is not to change anything or to feel different, relaxed, or calm; this may happen or it may not. Instead, the intention of the practice is, as best you can, to bring awareness to any sensations you feel as you focus your attention on each part of the body as I guide you through. If you find your mind wandering, which it inevitably will, gently just bringing it back to sensations in your body.

To begin, just notice your body lying or sitting here. What are the most obvious sensations? Maybe you notice touch or pressure where your body makes contact with the chair, the cushion, or the floor. Or an overall sense of temperature, or tension or relaxation. When you are ready, bringing your awareness to the physical sensations in your abdomen, becoming aware of the sensations there as you breathe in, and as you breathe out. Letting your body naturally breathe, and noticing what sensations are there. Taking a few minutes to feel these changing sensations.

Having connected with the sensations in the abdomen, we'll move the focus now down through the body, over to the left side, and into the left foot. Focusing just on the big toe of the left foot, as best you can. Seeing if you can connect with the actual sensations there, versus picturing that toe. Noticing anything that is happening in that toe. Maybe pulsing, or warmth. Or maybe you can feel the texture of a sock. Then allowing your focus to move to each of the toes of the left foot in turn, bringing a gentle curiosity to the quality of sensations you find, perhaps noticing the sense of contact between the toes, a sense of tingling, warmth, or no particular sensation. If there are areas you can't feel, that's okay. Just keeping your focus there, noticing whatever you can about that area.

When you are ready, letting go of awareness of the toes, and bringing your awareness to the sensations on the bottom of your left foot, bringing curiosity to the sole of the foot, tuning into any sensation there. Now bringing your attention to the top of the foot, then to the ankle. Feeling the muscles, bones, and tendons in the ankle. Now moving your attention

(continued)

46

up to the calf and the shin. Feeling the clothing against the skin of that area, or any sensations in the muscles. Now up into the knee. Detect as best you can all the sensations in these areas, sending your breath to each area as you move up the leg. You might think of your awareness as a spotlight, moving slowly through the body, bringing into focus any sensations in that area. Again, if there are areas where it is difficult to detect sensations, just feel as much as you can. Now bringing your attention to the left thigh. Noticing the sensations there. Maybe you feel the pressure of your leg against the chair, or places this part of the leg touches the floor if you are lying down.

Throughout this exercise, the mind will inevitably wander away from the breath and the body from time to time. That is entirely normal; it is what minds do. When you notice it, just acknowledge it, noticing where the mind has gone off to, and then gently return your attention to the part of the body.

Now sending your attention down to the right leg, through the right foot, and into the right toes. Continue to bring awareness, and gentle curiosity, to the physical sensations, allowing whatever sensations are in the toes to just be here as they are. Notice now what you feel in the bottom of your right foot, in the top of the foot, and the ankle. Bringing your awareness now up to your calf and noticing the sensations there. Now to the right knee.

If you feel any pain or discomfort in any of these areas, just be aware of it, your right thigh, noticing the sensations in this area. Maybe there is tightness in the muscle, or maybe you feel the pressure of this area against the chair, cushion, or floor. Then up into your hips and waist. Perhaps noticing the weight of the body against the chair (or the floor). Now moving your focus slowly up to your abdomen. Feeling it rising and falling with each breath. Now moving your awareness into your ribcage. Just feeling as many sensations as you can. Moving that spotlight of attention around to your back—the lower back, and the upper back, feeling the places where it touches the chair or the floor. Feeling any places of tension or discomfort. Now up into your chest and your shoulders.

If you notice your thoughts wandering, or if you become distracted or restless, just notice that too. It's okay. Just gently guide your attention back to the sensations in your body.

Guiding your attention now down the left arm and into the fingers of the left hand. Feeling each finger and maybe places where they contact the chair or your body. Now up into the wrist and forearm. Noticing all the sensations here. In the elbow, upper arm, the shoulder. Notice any tension, tightness.

Now gently moving your attention across your body to the right side, down the right arm, and into the fingers of the right hand. Feeling each of them separately. Maybe you notice tingling or urges to move them. Maybe there are fingers you are unable to feel as well as others. Now guiding your attention into the palm of the hand, and the wrist, the forearm and elbow. Now focusing on the upper arm and shoulder.

Gently let your attention now come into your neck. Feel where there is tightness or tension. Be aware of areas in which it is harder to detect sensation. Now bringing your focus up the back of your head. See if you can feel the hair on your head. Bringing awareness to the left ear, then over to the right ear. Now into the forehead.

Exploring now on the sensations in your face. Your eyes, your cheeks, your nose. See if you can feel the temperature of the breath and if that changes when you breathe in

(continued)

and out. Feeling any sensation in your lips, your chin, any tightness in your jaw. Bringing awareness to the very top of the head.

Now, after you have "scanned" the whole body in this way, spend a few minutes being aware of the body as a whole, and of the breath flowing freely in and out of the body.

Now very slowly and gently, while still maintaining an awareness of your body, when you are ready, maybe moving the body a little, wiggling the fingers and toes or gently stretching, then allowing your eyes to open, if they are closed, and your awareness to include the room, and the people around you.

Overview of Sessions
HANDOUT 1.1

SESSION 1: AUTOMATIC PILOT AND MINDFUL AWARENESS
In this first session, we discuss "automatic pilot," or the tendency to behave unconsciously or out of habit without full awareness of what we're doing. We discuss this specifically in relation to addictive behaviors (acting upon cravings and urges "automatically" without awareness). We introduce an exercise called the body scan to practice intentionally bringing attention to the body.

SESSION 2: A NEW RELATIONSHIP WITH DISCOMFORT
In this session, we learn ways to experience triggers and cravings without automatically reacting. We focus on recognizing triggers and what the reactions to those feel like, specifically the sensations, thoughts, and emotions that often accompany craving or reactivity. We use mindfulness to bring greater awareness to this often automatic process, learning to experience craving and urges in a way that increases our ability to make choices in how we respond.

SESSION 3: FROM REACTING TO RESPONDING
We learn the "SOBER space" as a way to expand our mindfulness skills from formal mindfulness practice to the daily situations we encounter. This may help us "be with" challenging physical sensations and emotions that arise, including those associated with cravings and urges, without reacting in harmful ways. We explore what might be driving these desires to use or react. In this session, we also learn formal sitting meditation.

SESSION 4: MINDFULNESS IN CHALLENGING SITUATIONS
We focus on being present in situations or with people previously associated with substance use or other reactive behaviors, using mindfulness to increase our ability to experience pressures or urges to use without automatically picking up a substance or reacting in other harmful ways. We identify our individual relapse risks and explore ways to cope with the intensity of feelings that come up in these high-risk situations.

SESSION 5: ACCEPTANCE AND SKILLFUL ACTION
It can often feel paradoxical to accept unwanted thoughts, feelings, and sensations as a way of moving through or past them. However, this may indeed be the first step in moving toward change. Acceptance of present experience is an important foundation for truly taking care of ourselves and seeing more clearly the best action to take. We continue to practice techniques such as the SOBER space and focus on using these in challenging situations. This session moves from noticing warning signs and learning to pause to taking skillful action in both high-risk situations and in normal daily life.

SESSION 6: SEEING THOUGHTS AS THOUGHTS
We further explore awareness of and relationship to thinking, with a focus on recognizing thoughts for what they are, versus assuming they are accurate reflections of the truth. We look at the role thoughts play in relapse cycles, specific thoughts that seem especially problematic, and ways to work more skillfully with our minds.

SESSION 7: SUPPORTING AND SUSTAINING WELL-BEING
This session focuses on personal warning signs for relapse and how to best respond when these warning signs arise. This includes discussion of broader lifestyle choices, balance, kindness toward ourselves and others, and the importance of including nourishing activities as part of a full, healthy life.

SESSION 8: SOCIAL SUPPORT AND CONTINUING PRACTICE
In this final session, we review skills and practices learned in this course and discuss the importance of building a support system. We reflect on what we learned from the course and share our individual plans for incorporating mindfulness practice into daily life.

THEME

"Automatic pilot" describes our tendency to react without awareness. When we experience cravings and urges to use substances, or engage in other reactive behaviors, we often go on automatic pilot; that is, we act upon urges without full awareness of what is happening and what the consequences might be. Practicing mindfulness can help us step out of this automatic pilot mode, raise our awareness, and make more conscious choices about how we respond rather than reacting in habitual and often self-defeating ways.

INTEGRATING PRACTICE INTO YOUR WEEK

1. Body Scan

Do your best to practice the body scan daily between now and when we meet again. There's no "right" way to do this nor is there anything in particular thing you "should" experience. Just notice whatever is arising in the present moment, including mind wandering, boredom, restlessness, sleepiness, and so forth.

2. Mindfulness of a Daily Activity

Choose an activity that you engage in each day (e.g., washing dishes, drinking coffee or tea) and, as best you can, bring your full attention to the experience in the same way we did with the raisin. You may notice qualities of the object or activity as well as sensations, thoughts, or feelings that arise.

3. Complete Daily Practice Tracking Sheet

Fill this out daily, recording your mindfulness practice (both the body scan and mindfulness of a daily activity) and what you noticed or what got in the way. Please be honest. You will not be judged in any way about how much or how little you have integrated practices each week, or about your experiences.

Daily Practice Tracking Sheet
HANDOUT 1.3

Instructions: Each day, record your mindfulness practice, also noting any barriers, observations, or comments.

Day/date	Formal practice with audio recording: How long?	Mindfulness of daily activities	Observations/comments
	____ minutes	What activities?	
	____ minutes	What activities?	
	____ minutes	What activities?	
	____ minutes	What activities?	
	____ minutes	What activities?	
	____ minutes	What activities?	
	____ minutes	What activities?	

A New Relationship with Discomfort

Pain is inevitable, suffering is optional.
—BUDDHA

Materials

- Bell
- Whiteboard/markers
- Handout 2.1: Common Challenges in Meditation Practice (and in Daily Life)
- Handout 2.2: Noticing Triggers Worksheet
- Handout 2.3: Session 2 Theme and Daily Practice: A New Relationship with Discomfort
- Handout 2.4: Daily Practice Tracking Sheet
- Audio Files: Body Scan, Urge Surfing, Mountain Meditation

Theme

This session focuses on recognizing triggers, and on experiencing them without automatically reacting. We begin by learning to identify triggers, and we observe how they often lead to a chain of sensations, thoughts, emotions, and behaviors. Mindfulness can bring this process into awareness, disrupting automatic reactive behaviors and allowing greater flexibility and choice.

Goals

- Continue to practice awareness of body sensations.
- Bring awareness to physical sensations, thoughts and emotions in reaction to triggers.

- Explore how these experiences can lead to a chain of habitual, reactive behaviors, and can cause us to lose our present-moment awareness.

- Introduce mindful awareness as a way to create a "pause" in this typically automatic process.

Session Outline

- Check-In
- Body Scan (Practice 1.2)
- Home Practice Review and Common Challenges
- Walking Down the Street Exercise (Practice 2.1)
- Urge Surfing (Practice 2.2) and Discussion of Craving
- Mountain Meditation (Practice 2.3)
- Daily Practice
- Closing

Practice for This Week

- Body scan
- Daily Practice Tracking Sheet
- Noticing Triggers Worksheet
- Mindfulness of a daily activity

CHECK-IN

Facilitators may wish to start with a brief one- to two-word check-in ("Name one or two things you notice—a physical sensation, thought or mind state, or an emotion that you observe in this moment"). This is best kept brief. It can help for the facilitator to model this (e.g., "relaxed and excited" or "chilly feet").

BODY SCAN

Starting in this second week, each session begins with a 20- to 30-minute formal mindfulness practice, followed by inquiry about experiences during the practice. Beginning with formal practice at the start of each session, prior to any discussion, reinforces the experiential nature of the course. The body scan practice from Session 1 (Practice 1.2) is practiced again at the start of Session 2.

HOME PRACTICE REVIEW AND COMMON CHALLENGES

By Session 2, participants have experienced their first week of practicing the body scan meditation on their own using the audio recording and have typically already begun to encounter some challenges. Thus, one objective of this session is to acknowledge and discuss these challenges, address concerns and questions, and clarify misconceptions about meditation. The format and style of this discussion are similar to those described in the previous session, reflecting a sense of curiosity and nonjudgment about whatever experiences participants offer. Some of the most common issues that arise in practice are physical discomfort, drowsiness and sleepiness, feelings of restlessness, self-judgment, and expectations about the practice creating a sense of peace and relaxation.

These challenges reflect those described in traditional Buddhist teachings. Although it is not necessary (nor recommended) that facilitators refer to Buddhist terminology in MBRP, this framework can be a useful way to identify the challenges that often arise for practitioners of mindfulness meditation (Handout 2.1). Traditional mindfulness meditation teachings describe five categories of challenges (or "hindrances"): (1) "aversion," which could include fear, anger, irritation, resentment, and all of their varied forms; (2) "craving and desire," or the experience of wanting, which may be as subtle as wanting to feel relaxed and peaceful and as extreme as an intense urge to use a substance; (3) "restlessness and agitation," which may be experienced physically, as a strong desire to move, or as mental agitation; (4) "drowsiness or fogginess," which may be in the form of sleepiness, mental sluggishness, or lethargy; and (5) "doubt," which may be personal doubt, or doubt about the practice and its purpose or utility.

A common experience when these states arise is for a meditator to attempt to get rid of them so that she or he can reengage in the meditation, believing that these experiences are problems that are getting in the way of practice. Although there are skillful ways to work with these states, observing them *is part of meditation practice,* just as observing body states is part of the body scan practice. We are learning to recognize these states and cultivate a curious attitude about them, rather than resist or attempt to eradicate them.

Aversion

The first opportunity to work with aversion often arises in the form of physical discomfort. By the end of this first week of practice, participants may have become more acutely aware of both the sensations of discomfort in the body and their reactions to these sensations. Irritation, self-judgment, and a desire to "fix" or "get rid of" the discomfort are common. Participants may also experience confusion, doubt, and disappointment about mindfulness practice based on prior assumptions and expectations about the "pleasant" or "blissful" experiences that should accompany meditation. There is often a need for repeated emphasis on the purpose or intention of these practices, especially in beginning sessions. In this second week, we emphasize increasing awareness and acceptance of all phenomena, including uncomfortable or unwanted experiences, as well as reactions to these phenomena. We also inquire about some of these experiences, regardless of whether participants voluntarily raise them in discussion, emphasizing that no experience is "right" or "better" than any other. Failing to address these experiences may leave participants feeling as though they "don't get it" or "aren't doing it right."

PARTICIPANT 1: I was really distracted by an itch on my knee and couldn't focus on the instructions. I was trying to ignore the itch, but my mind kept going back to it.

FACILITATOR: What did the itch feel like?

PARTICIPANT 1: It was annoying. I wanted to scratch it.

FACILITATOR: So you noticed the itch, then some annoyance, and an urge to scratch the itch. What did the urge feel like?

PARTICIPANT 1: Like restlessness. I felt like it was getting in the way of my doing the exercise.

FACILITATOR: Was there a thought?

PARTICIPANT 1: Yes, I thought, "This is getting in my way. I can't concentrate."

PARTICIPANT 2: I felt the same way about the tension in my back.

FACILITATOR: Okay, great—thank you. This is a common experience: some discomfort arises, and then a desire to make it go away. The thing about this practice is we get to bring attention and curiosity to whatever is happening, even if it's something we didn't necessarily want or expect. Just noticing, what does an itch really feel like? Is it tingling? Is it hot? Of course, you can scratch or shift positions if you need to, but just noticing it for a moment before you do that, instead of immediately reacting as we usually do—why do you think we might want to do that?

PARTICIPANT 3: I don't know. Why would I want to be with something uncomfortable, especially if I can make it go away really easily?

FACILITATOR: Right, most of us don't want to feel discomfort. So what might be the value of practicing staying with it?

PARTICIPANT 1: Not just reacting automatically, I guess.

FACILITATOR: So to practice pausing before reacting. How do you think this might be useful in your life?

PARTICIPANT 1: Well, when I have a craving, I usually react just automatically without really thinking about it. Like scratching an itch.

FACILITATOR: Yes. Other thoughts?

PARTICIPANT 2: Avoiding pain is one of my biggest reasons for using. Not just physical pain, but also emotional pain. And look where that got me. The avoiding just doesn't work. Or I guess it works for a brief period, but then makes it worse.

FACILITATOR: In a way it gives the pain more power, doesn't it? And sometimes the struggle against pain is worse than the pain itself. This isn't about punishing ourselves by sitting with pain; we're practicing bringing gentleness to it, making space for it, so that we have some freedom and we can change our relationship to it and respond in the way we'd really like to.

Here the facilitator introduces the idea of becoming aware of sensations of discomfort as simply another phenomenon that is occurring in the present moment and reminds the group that the idea of the practice is not just remaining focused on the breath to the exclusion of all other experience, but noticing and becoming curious about all phenomena, including discomfort. The facilitator ties this into the experience of craving and our tendency to react automatically. The facilitator also emphasizes that mindfulness is not necessarily about changing one's experience, but about creating a different relationship to it. This includes creating space for difficult experiences, which may help participants begin to discover that what is so painful is sometimes not the sensation or feeling itself, but the aversion to it or ongoing attempts to control it.

Craving and Desire

The challenge of craving or desire often arises in the form of a longing for peacefulness or relaxation. It is a common belief among beginning mindfulness practitioners that deep concentration and bliss mean "good" practice and anything less is "bad" or "not working." It's easy for meditators to feel that something is wrong with their practice when they notice they have been repeatedly distracted. Similarly, many beginning meditators come with the idea that the purpose is relaxation, and they expect immediate freedom from stress, struggle, and discomfort. They are often disappointed when practice does not immediately bring about these states. Thus, it is helpful to remind participants that we practice to increase our awareness and to develop a spacious, nonjudgmental attitude toward all experience, including discomfort, distraction, or stress. Experiences of peace or relaxation are explored in the same way that discomfort might be, with careful attention to any misconceptions that these states are the goal of practice.

PARTICIPANT 1: I found this practice very relaxing.

FACILITATOR: Okay. Were there particular sensations you noticed in your body?

PARTICIPANT 1: Just a feeling of ease. I was also less anxious. I noticed my mind wasn't wandering as much. It really worked this time.

FACILITATOR: What do you mean when you say it "worked"?

PARTICIPANT 1: I felt calmer. Usually my mind is just all over the place, and that is one of my biggest triggers for drinking. Just coming back to what is actually going on in the moment. I was really surprised by how well it worked.

FACILITATOR: So you noticed that your mind wasn't wandering quite as much and that you were feeling calmer.

PARTICIPANT 1: Yes.

FACILITATOR: And it sounds like you believed this meant it was "working." Do you think it will always be relaxing when you meditate?

PARTICIPANT 1: (*laughs*) No, probably not.

FACILITATOR: It sounds like a very pleasant experience. And it is also helpful to remember that every time you do it, it is different. Sometimes you might find yourself feeling peaceful and relaxed and experiencing all these pleasant sensations, other times you might feel sleepy or restless or agitated. This does not mean that the meditation is "not working" or that we are doing something wrong. It is simply what's happening, and we are practicing being more aware of it, and maybe a little less reactive.

Restlessness and Agitation

Restlessness is a common experience in meditation, experienced both physically and mentally (e.g., racing thoughts, excessive planning or rumination). As with all these challenges, we turn attention toward the experience rather than attempt to suppress or control it. One might begin by acknowledging its presence and approaching it with curiosity, perhaps noticing where it lives in the body and if there is any reaction to the experience.

PARTICIPANT 1: I got tired of the repetition in the audio recording, hearing the same thing over and over again. I noticed that at one point last night I got really agitated. So I just turned it off.

FACILITATOR: Okay, interesting! What did the agitation feel like?

PARTICIPANT 1: Just restless and like, "When will this end? I just want to turn it off."

FACILITATOR: So it sounds like there were some sensations in the body, and also the thought "I want to turn this off"? If you all remember what we talked about last time: Whatever comes up is part of your mindfulness practice. That includes the agitation, the thoughts, the urge to act on thoughts, all of this. It may be interesting to check that out for a bit: the experience of agitation and the sensations and thoughts that go along with it, even just an extra moment or two. What else did people notice?

PARTICIPANT 2: Sometimes when I am practicing, I find that my mind gets caught in thinking about the instructions . . . why is she saying this or that, why is there such a long pause, what's coming next? And then I catch myself and try and come back to the practice.

FACILITATOR: So you noticed the mind getting caught up in questioning or analyzing, and then you guided your attention back. When that happened, was there any judgment?

PARTICIPANT 2: Yeah, like, "Come on, there you go, overanalyzing things again."

FACILITATOR: Okay. Did you notice any emotion?

PARTICIPANT 2: Yeah, some frustration.

FACILITATOR: All right, thank you. Again, and we will return to this repeatedly throughout the course, the idea here is not to get rid of the thoughts or even judgment that comes up. We're not fighting or getting rid of anything. We're just pausing and noticing, becoming aware of whatever is going on. So when you find yourself going into analyzing or creating a story about what's happening, the moment you become aware of that, that's a moment of mindfulness. Each time you become aware, simply letting go and beginning again . . . without forcing or struggling, even if you have to do this over and over again. And if you become aware of struggle, just noticing that with the same gentle attention, letting go of that, starting again.

Drowsiness/Sleepiness

Drowsiness is another common experience in meditation practice, particularly in the body scan, which often involves lying down with eyes closed. This may be in part just the natural response of the body to settling down and taking a break from the hectic pace of our lives. However, sleepiness and drowsiness can be included in our attention. One might observe the experience of drowsiness itself: What does it feel like? Is it possible to pay attention to the moments when we are startled into wakefulness? What is the mind's reaction to feeling sleepy? Is there self-judgment? If sleepiness is persistent, we might also offer suggestions for ways to work with this mind state.

> PARTICIPANT: I made the mistake of doing the body scan in my bedroom and I fell asleep.
>
> FACILITATOR: What was your response when you noticed you'd fallen asleep?
>
> PARTICIPANT: Well, at first, it was fine because it was just relaxing, but when it happened a few times I got frustrated with myself.
>
> FACILITATOR: Do you remember any thoughts or physical experiences that went with that frustration? How did you know you were experiencing frustration?
>
> PARTICIPANT: Just kind of a feeling of agitation and feeling like I'm not listening to the instructions.
>
> FACILITATOR: So a physical feeling of agitation and the thought, like, "I'm not listening to the instructions"?
>
> PARTICIPANT: Yeah.
>
> FACILITATOR: What do you think it would be like to just bring curiosity to the experience of frustration, to that drowsiness right before you fall asleep, or the startled response when you first wake up, noticing the thoughts that go through your mind and the emotional and physical feeling of frustration?
>
> PARTICIPANT: I don't know. I usually try to fix it or just get frustrated.
>
> FACILITATOR: It's possible to make all of that part of your practice; in fact, it *is* your practice in that moment because this is what is happening. We are practicing observing whatever our experience is with curiosity, a more open and relaxed awareness, and without judgment of this experience as "right" or "wrong." Just letting it be what it is. You might play with that this coming week.
>
> If you notice sleepiness happening over and over again, though, it might be helpful to sit up straight and be in a more alert posture. You could even practice in a standing posture. You can also keep your eyes open while you are practicing to let some light in, or try practicing at a different time of day. Just experiment with it and see what happens.

Once again, the facilitator draws attention to observing the present moment, including the experience of sleepiness, and encourages curiosity about both its qualities and the mind's reaction to it (e.g., self-judgment, irritation, frustration). She also offers ways to work with it if it repeatedly arises.

Doubt

As stated earlier, doubt may express itself in different forms, including doubt about the practice itself and/or about one's ability to engage in it. Self-judgment is a particularly common manifestation of both aversion and doubt in these beginning stages of meditation. It often accompanies, or is experienced as, a reaction to one of the other challenges such as sleepiness, restlessness, or discomfort. It may also occur in reaction to a thought, sensation, or emotional state. We find it useful to repeatedly inquire about experiences of judgment, particularly in response to anything challenging or unpleasant that arises (e.g., sleepiness, pain, or anger). Inquiring about doubt or self-judgment not only encourages greater awareness but conveys a wider, gentler, more compassionate stance toward oneself and one's experience. It is also an opportunity for participants to recognize the universality of these experiences as they hear it reflected in the comments of their fellow group members.

WALKING DOWN THE STREET EXERCISE

The intention of this exercise (Practice 2.1) is to allow participants to observe the initial, often habitual, response of the mind to an ambiguous stimulus, and to identify the cascade of thoughts, emotions, physical sensations, and urges that follow. The scenario is purposely very simple and intended to be presented briefly. *It is important to leave the key stimulus ambiguous*; that is, the failure of the imagined person in the scenario to return the greeting should be presented with a neutral tone and language so the facilitator does not suggest any explanation for the behavior (i.e., "the person just continues to walk by and does not wave back"). This allows the mind to project its own story onto the situation.

Following the exercise, participants are invited to describe any thoughts that went through their minds and any feelings, sensations, or urges to react. It may be helpful to list these on the whiteboard. We often use columns to differentiate thoughts, physical sensations, emotions, and urges, and to illustrate the ways these experiences affect one another (e.g., a thought eliciting a feeling). As discussed previously, we sometimes inquire whether the reaction is familiar, encouraging participants to begin recognizing patterns of thoughts, assumptions, or reactions when encountering triggers or situations that may be unclear or unsettling in some way.

This exercise also allows participants to see the varying interpretations one can make of the same event, and to recognize these as "interpretations" or stories rather than "facts." Being able to recognize and label reactions in this way may help increase awareness of habitual reactions and create a pause in the seemingly automatic chain of experiences. We also use this exercise as preparation for the next practice, which involves becoming aware of one's thoughts, feelings, and sensations in a situation that may be more challenging and can elicit cravings and urges.

> FACILITATOR: What did people notice in that exercise? We don't need to know about the person or the situation—I am curious about what you noticed about your reactions. [Facilitator notes experiences in separate columns on the whiteboard—thoughts/sensations/emotions/urges—as participants share.]

> PARTICIPANT 1: I felt anxious.

> FACILITATOR: Okay, and was there a thought associated with that feeling? What happened first, if you recall?

> PARTICIPANT 1: First, I felt excited to see him. Then when he didn't wave, I thought, "Why isn't he saying hello to me?" and I felt anxious.

> FACILITATOR: So you felt excitement when you first saw him, then had the thought "Why isn't he saying hello?." What did the excitement feel like, do you remember?

> PARTICIPANT 1: Kind of a light feeling, especially in my upper body.

> FACILITATOR: Lightness, and then when he didn't wave, you had a thought like "Why isn't he saying hello?" and a feeling of anxiety. Is that right?

> PARTICIPANT 1: Yes.

> FACILITATOR: So how did you experience the anxiety? Were there thoughts? Sensations in the body?

> PARTICIPANT 1: It wasn't physical; it was more mental . . . racing thoughts in my mind, and "Why didn't he wave back? Did he not see me?" or maybe it was personal, like maybe I did something.

> FACILITATOR: It sounds like there was some self-doubt in there, an assumption that you had done something wrong. Is this reaction familiar?

> PARTICIPANT 1: Yeah, it is. I tend to assume that when things go wrong, it's my fault.

> FACILITATOR: Okay. Did you notice any urges to react in a certain way?

> PARTICIPANT 1: Yeah, I wanted to go home. Isolate.

> FACILITATOR: Thank you for sharing that—anyone else have a similar or maybe different experience?

PARTICIPANT 2: I went after him, yelling to get his attention.

FACILITATOR: Okay. Do you remember right before you went after him what you felt or thought?

PARTICIPANT 2: Confusion, then the thought "Did he not see me?" Then this urge to run after him, to fix it.

FACILITATOR: So feeling confusion, then a thought, then an urge. Did you notice any sensations that went along with the urge?

PARTICIPANT 2: I noticed my breathing change. It got a little quicker, sort of more abrupt.

The facilitator might ask for a few more examples, using the whiteboard to list thoughts, physical sensations, emotions, and urges in separate columns. This may help participants begin to make these distinctions themselves, teasing apart the seemingly automatic and often overwhelming flood of experience. They may also begin to see how thoughts, feelings, sensations, and urges can proliferate, triggering one another.

FACILITATOR: So you can see here the range of different responses to the same event. Which one is correct? [Participants often comment that no one interpretation is "right."] There isn't right or wrong, is there? All just interpretation and reaction. Why might it be important to bring more awareness to these reactions? [The discussion might refer back to the previous week's discussion of stepping out of automatic ways of reacting, giving ourselves more freedom to make purposeful choices.]

When people are asked what they learned from the exercise, they often comment that they recognize how their interpretations of an event affect their thoughts and emotions and how automatic this process often seems. They also begin to recognize how their interpretations may not be reflective of the truth and may cause them undue distress or lead to reactive behavior. This exercise lays the foundation for the following exercise in which participants are asked to pay attention to the same type of reactivity in a more challenging situation.

URGE SURFING AND DISCUSSION OF CRAVING

This practice (Practice 2.2) is designed to shift the relationship to experiences of cravings or urges to react unskillfully (e.g., use substances) from one of fear or resistance to that of "being with" in a curious and kind way. The exercise invites participants to explore the many elements of craving or urges, observing first the physical sensations as well as the accompanying thoughts and urges, dismantling an often overwhelming experience that might typically elicit reactivity, feelings of defeat or fear, or attempts to control the experience. Participants practice a curious, compassionate approach versus a habitual or automatic reaction. They are invited to look "underneath" or "behind" the craving; underlying the overwhelming desire for a substance is often a deeper need—perhaps relief from challenging emotions or a desire for joy, peace, or freedom.

Participants are encouraged to choose a reasonable scenario for this exercise, that is, something that has been challenging or stressful but perhaps not the most challenging situation in their lives or their biggest trigger. We often suggest that on a scale from 1 to 10, with 10 being the hardest thing they experience, they choose something around a 3 or 4. They are first asked to picture this challenging situation right up until the point at which they would typically react in some way, and then pause and observe thoughts, feelings, and bodily sensations rather than immediately falling into familiar patterns or reactive behavior. It is suggested that they bring a similar exploration and curiosity to this experience as they did with the raisin or to bodily sensations in the body scan. In many ways, this practice encompasses the core of the MBRP approach; we practice recognizing both the discomfort and the accompanying reactions, including urges to escape it or change an unwanted experience. Then, rather than falling into immediate reaction or resisting the experience, we practice pausing and observing what the urge actually feels like. We then practice approaching this experience with gentle, nonjudgmental curiosity rather than defaulting to habitual reactive behaviors.

The "urge surfing" is introduced as a metaphor to illustrate the possibility of staying present with the intensity of an urge without becoming subsumed or behaving reactively. Participants are asked to picture the urge as an ocean wave and imagine themselves surfing, using their breath as a surfboard to ride the wave. They are staying in contact with the experience but are not subsumed by it. They are able to balance, and they ride the wave through its peak and its decline. We have found that although some participants find this visualization helpful in relating differently to urges, others have difficulty with either visualization or staying present with the intensity of an urge or craving. We thus present it as simply one option with which to experiment and have encouraged participants to alter and change the metaphor to suit their individual needs. The primary intention in using the metaphor is to convey the possibility of observing urges and cravings without having to act upon or fight them. This practice not only reveals the impermanent nature of craving, but it also increases participants' confidence in their ability to experience discomfort and stay present with intensity.

The practice instructions also include a suggestion that participants ask themselves, "What do I really need in this situation?" Craving or urges to react in response to a trigger can, at times, be primarily physiological. However, they may also mask another emotional state (e.g., loneliness, hurt, resentment, or feelings of betrayal) with an intense desire to alleviate the discomfort. It may be a sign that our needs are not being met. When cravings or urges arise, it is sometimes helpful to investigate a little further what is really wanted or needed. We find, of course, that it is seldom the thing we are reaching for. The object of desire may be a poor substitute that satisfies us for a moment but inevitably leaves a deeper dissatisfaction in its wake, intensifying the future cycle of desire.

We begin inquiry by asking what specific physical sensations, thoughts, and emotions arose for people in this scenario, specifying that we are not so much interested in the scenario itself, but in what they noticed about their experience. We inquire whether there were emotions or sensations that felt intolerable, or urges to escape the experience. Maybe this was accompanied by a thought or belief that they "couldn't stand it" or needed to "fix" it. This can help develop a curiosity about the experience, learning to relate to craving differently, perhaps even with curiosity. At this point, however, the main intention of the exercise is to offer an experiential understanding of "being with" the urge or craving rather than "giving in" to it.

Following some inquiry about experiences, it can be helpful to illustrate on the whiteboard the theory behind urge surfing (see Figure 2.1). When a craving begins, it might feel as though its intensity will continue to grow until we act on it (left-hand graph). However, if we wait it out, the craving may naturally ebb and flow, like a wave (right-hand graph). Eventually, it will subside.

> FACILITATOR: Most of us have the idea that once craving or urges begin and there is that impulse to react, the intensity of it will continue to increase until we act on it or stop it somehow. We often imagine craving as a straight line continuing upward until we alleviate it by using (*drawing diagonal line sloping upward on the whiteboard*). In reality, craving is typically less like a line and more like a wave; it ebbs to a peak, and then, if we wait it out, it

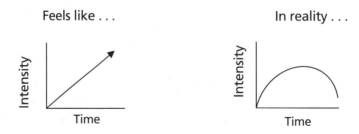

FIGURE 2.1. The theory behind urge surfing.

will naturally subside (*drawing a line rising, reaching a plateau, then falling, like a wave*).

One way to get rid of an urge or craving is to engage in a behavior, such as substance use, in response to it. We might feel relief or happiness for a while, but this is a little like trying to quench thirst by drinking salt water: you are temporarily relieved, but then you are left even thirstier than you were to begin with. Attempting to fight the craving might be another way we try to control it. However, when cravings and urges are suppressed, they often just get stronger. So what happens if instead of trying to get rid of or suppress it, we just stay with it without reacting?

As we keep practicing this surfing, the intensity of the urge or craving tends to decrease a little bit (*drawing shallower curves*), and we get better at waiting it out and become more confident that we are able to ride this wave without getting wiped out.

PARTICIPANT: Maybe that would work to wait it out once, but then the craving just comes back again.

FACILITATOR: Sure, it probably will come back. And if you used alcohol or a drug to make it go away, wouldn't it come back too? Cravings might arise and pass many times in one day, and this way of being with the experience, or "surfing," may need to be practiced over and over again. It does get a little easier, and the cravings often become less intense because you're not feeding them or fighting them. Whereas when we use in response to the craving, we're feeding it, making it stronger, and when we attempt to fight it, we often wear ourselves down and are more likely to feel defeated and want to give up.

There's often the thought or belief "I can't do this." And we're learning that we are able to do this differently, but it takes practice. You've just done it here; you experienced craving or an urge and successfully stayed present without acting on it. Maybe it wasn't as intense as what you might encounter in the future, but just like when you are first learning to surf, you ride small waves first, you practice. Once those become easier, then you can take on bigger ones.

MOUNTAIN MEDITATION

The previous urge surfing practice sometimes elicits challenging experiences or arousal. We thus conclude the session with a stabilizing and grounding practice. We typically use the Mountain Meditation guided practice (Practice 2.3) adapted from a practice used by Jon Kabat-Zinn (1994). The meditation involves visualizing a mountain and calling to mind qualities of stability, strength, and dignity. Participants are asked to imagine merging with this image of the mountain, embodying these qualities as their own and experiencing a sense of poise and solidity, even in the face of changing circumstances, situations, and inner states. We have found that most participants respond favorably to this metaphor and have little trouble imagining qualities of strength and constancy. However, some express discomfort or difficulty imagining themselves as the mountain, either feeling incapable of experiencing such strength and solidity or having trouble with the visualization. Just as with any other practice, we encourage a gentle, kind awareness of the reactions that arise. It may also be useful to play with the metaphor, modifying it as needed. Picturing the mountain is just a vehicle to contact an experience of the qualities it holds, and to recognize these same qualities in ourselves. For those with difficulties visualizing, they might let go of efforts to find an image and instead simply invite in the qualities of rootedness, dignity, and strength.

PRACTICE FOR THIS WEEK

In addition to continuing daily practice of the body scan and engaging mindfully in a daily activity, participants are asked to use the Noticing Triggers Worksheet (Handout 2.2) to log triggers they encounter over the upcoming week and note any subsequent thoughts, emotions, and physical reactions (Handout 2.3). They are also asked to describe behaviors they engage in to cope with the experience. The purpose of this worksheet is to bring both the triggers and reactions into fuller awareness and to continue the practice of differentiating among thoughts, feelings, and bodily sensations. The intention is *not* to track whether the reaction was "good" or "bad," but rather to notice habitual or "automatic" reactions. Participants also complete the Daily Practice Tracking Sheet (Handout 2.4) to supplement their awareness of what they are learning and to give facilitators insight into any concerns or barriers.

CLOSING

Although we have found that typically by the end of the session any anxiety or craving participants experience during the urge surfing exercise has waned, we invite them to briefly state one to two words describing how they are feeling (sensation, mind state, or emotion). Again, it can be helpful for facilitators to model this by offering an observation of their own experience in the same one- to two-word format.

Walking Down the Street Exercise
PRACTICE 2.1

Intentions

+ Observing the tendency for proliferation of thoughts, emotions, physical sensations, and urges to react in response to the *interpretation of* an ambiguous event

+ Seeing the varying interpretations and recognizing them as such, rather than as the "truth"

+ Beginning to differentiate thoughts, emotions, physical sensations, and urges and noticing how they affect (or "feed") one another

+ Noticing if reactions are familiar, thus beginning to recognize patterns in response to triggers

We are constantly interpreting and judging our experience. These stories and judgments often proliferate, leading to further thoughts, sensations, emotional states, and sometimes urges to react. We might find ourselves in an emotional state or engaging in a behavior with little awareness of how we got there. Here we use a simple example to illustrate this.

Find a comfortable position in your chair. Allow your eyes to close, if you choose, and take a moment to just settle in. I am going to ask you to imagine a simple scenario and to just notice as much as you can about your thoughts, emotions, and body sensations. Imagine now that you are walking down the street. Picture a familiar location, and really see the sights around you, hear the sounds that might be in this area, maybe cars, birds, people's voices. Or maybe it's very quiet. Now imagine that you see someone you know on the other side of the street, walking in the opposite direction, so the person is coming toward you. Let this be someone you are happy to see—maybe a friend, a coworker, or anyone you might want to say hello to. Picture that person now. As you see this person walking toward you, notice what thoughts are going through your mind and any emotions or sensations you may be experiencing.

As the person comes toward you, you smile and wave. But the person does not wave back and just continues to walk by.

Notice now what is going through your mind. What thoughts are arising? Notice any sensations in your body. And what feelings or emotions are present? Notice if you have an urge to act in a particular way.

When you are ready, allow this scenario to fade and gently bring your awareness back into the room and allow your eyes to open.

Adapted from Segal, Williams, and Teasdale (2013). Copyright © 2013 The Guilford Press. Used by permission.

Urge Surfing Exercise
PRACTICE 2.2

Intentions

✦ Exposure/response prevention: staying present with and observing the experience of craving/urges with kindness and curiosity, without engaging in reactive or resistant behavior

✦ Exploring the experience of craving, including physical sensations, thoughts, and urges, to dismantle an experience that often feels overwhelming and typically elicits reactivity

✦ Looking "beneath" the craving for underlying, often wholesome, needs (e.g., relief from difficult emotions, a desire for peace or freedom)

Now we'll do a practice similar to the last one, but this time instead of giving you a scenario to imagine, I'll ask you to picture a situation that you find challenging in your present life, one in which you are triggered in some way. This might be a situation that in the past caused urges to be reactive, maybe in a way that is not in line with how you want to be in your life. Please take care of yourself by choosing something that is challenging but not overwhelming. On a scale from 1 to 10, where 10 is the hardest thing you experience, maybe about a 3. Anyone need another moment to come up with something?

As you picture this scene from your life, I will ask you to imagine that you do *not* engage in the reactive behavior, whatever that might be for you. I'll encourage you to bring yourself right up to the point of reactivity, where you might be tempted to engage in the behavior, but to pause right there and not go beyond that point. We'll pause there and explore that experience. If the scenario you pick feels overwhelming, like something you are not ready to work with right now, or if you find yourself going beyond the point where you can maintain awareness and curiosity and becoming flooded by the experience, please respect this limit and honor yourself by grounding in the present moment, opening your eyes, returning to your breath if that is a safe anchor for you, standing up, moving a little, or focusing on your physical surroundings (it may be helpful here to refer to the zones of engagement).

Do you all have a situation in mind? Does anyone need another minute to come up with something?

Now close your eyes, if that feels comfortable. You may also leave them open if you choose, maintaining a soft focus a few feet in front of you and letting your gaze just rest there throughout the exercise. Take a few moments to just feel your body here in the chair (or on the cushion). Noticing sensations. Letting the breath flow easily in and out. Now bringing this scenario you've chosen to mind, taking the time you need to really picture yourself in that place or situation, or maybe with that person if there's someone else involved. Now begin to let the scene play out—imagining the events or situation that lead up to this point of reactivity. Maybe someone says or does something that triggers you, or something happens around you. Now we're just going to pause for a moment right here before the reaction comes and explore our experience a little, finding a balance, just staying with and observing the experience without reacting.

So you might begin by noticing any physical sensations that are arising. What does

(continued)

68

this feel like in your body? Then noticing what thoughts might be going through your mind. Or maybe the mind feels scattered or blank. Now observing what emotions you are experiencing in this situation. Maybe there is a predominant one, or maybe there are several emotions. Noticing, too, what it is about this experience that feels intolerable. Can you stay with it, and be gentle with yourself? If you begin to feel overwhelmed at any point, you can always back off a bit by allowing your eyes to open or letting your attention come back to observing your breathing. Remember that we are practicing staying with this experience in a kind, curious way. We are pausing here to observe, as best we can, what is happening in the body and mind, what this craving or urge *feels* like.

If this urge becomes increasingly intense, you might imagine it as an ocean wave . . . imagine that you are riding that wave, using your breath as a surfboard to stay steady. . . . Your job is to ride the wave from its beginning, as it grows, staying right with it, through the peak of its intensity, keeping your balance while the wave rises and staying on top of it until it naturally begins to subside. You are staying in contact with this experience, riding on top of rather than succumbing to it or being wiped out by it. Just observing as the intensity rises and falls, and trusting that without any action on your part, this wave will rise and then it will fall, and eventually begin to fade.

Noticing now how you can simply stay present with this wave instead of immediately reacting to it, without giving in to the urge, without acting on it, without having to make it go away.

As you stay with this experience, asking yourself the question "What is it I *really* need in this situation?" You don't need to find an answer—just ask yourself the question and see what you notice.

Now, taking the time you need, gently letting go of the scenario you've imagined, and slowly and gently bringing your attention back to your body sitting here in this room. Taking a deep breath if you'd like to. Maybe moving the body a little if that feels right. Opening your eyes and taking in the room and people around you.

Mountain Meditation
PRACTICE 2.3

Intentions

✦ Embodying the stabilizing, grounded, rooted, and still qualities of a mountain, even in the face of inner and outer "weather" (e.g., changing circumstances, challenging situations or emotions)

✦ Knowing that we have these inner resources available to us at any time

---

Settle into a comfortable position, with your spine straight but relaxed, and your head balanced easily on your neck and shoulders, sitting with a sense of dignity and ease. Letting your body support the intention to remain wakeful and present. You might allow your eyes to close if that is comfortable for you, or allow them to rest in a soft gaze, perhaps a few feet in front of you on the floor. And now bringing your attention to rest on the sensation of the breath as it naturally flows in and out of the body. Observing the feel of your body breathing. Coming into stillness, sitting with a sense of completeness, with your posture reflecting this.

Now, when you are ready, bringing to mind an image of a mountain. Picturing the most beautiful mountain you can imagine, and allowing this mountain to come more clearly into view. If picturing a mountain is difficult, imagining the qualities of a mountain and coming into contact with the felt sense of these qualities, including the rootedness, the massiveness and solidity. Noticing how unmoving it is, how beautiful in its own unique shape and form. Maybe your mountain has snow or trees on it. Perhaps it has one prominent peak, or several. However it appears, just sitting and breathing with the image of this mountain, observing its qualities.

And when you're ready, seeing if you can bring the mountain into your body so that your body sitting here and the mountain in your mind's eye become one. So that as you sit here, you become the mountain. Your head becomes the mountain's peak, your shoulders and arms the sides of the mountain, your hips and legs the solid base rooted to your cushion or your chair. Experiencing in your body a sense of uplift from the base of the mountain up through your spine. With each breath, becoming more and more a living, breathing mountain, unwavering in your stillness, complete, centered, rooted, and majestic.

Through periods of light and dark, changes in seasons and in weather, the mountain just sits. At times it may find itself covered by fog or pelted by rain. People may come to see the mountain and be disappointed if they can't see it clearly or if it's not what they expected it to be, or they may comment on how beautiful it is, or they may disrespect or ignore it. And through all this, the mountain just sits. Solid and steady. At times visited by powerful storms, snow, rain, and winds of unthinkable magnitude; through it all the mountain just sits, unmoved by what happens on the surface.

As we sit holding this image or these qualities in our mind, we can embody the same unwavering stillness and rootedness in the face of everything that changes in our own lives, over seconds, hours, days, and years. In our meditation practice and in our lives, we experience the constant change all around us and in our own minds and bodies.

We have our own periods of light and dark. We experience clouds and storms. We endure periods of darkness and pain as well as moments of joy. People sometimes appreciate and other times criticize us. Even our appearance changes constantly, like the mountain's, experiencing a weathering of its own.

By being our own kind of mountain in our meditation, we can tune in to these qualities of strength and stability that we already have inside of us.

In the last moments of this practice, continue to sit with this image of the mountain, embodying its rootedness, stillness, and majesty, until you hear the sound of the bell.

Adapted from Kabat-Zinn (1994). Copyright © 1994 Jon Kabat-Zinn. Used by permission.

Common Challenges in Meditation Practice (and in Daily Life)

HANDOUT 2.1

There are some challenges that arise so commonly in the course of meditation practice that this list has remained steady over thousands of years. These experiences are not bad or wrong; they are simply part of meditation practice, and they do not mean that your meditation is "not working" or that you are doing the practice incorrectly. These challenges can feel distracting, and people often feel defeated or discouraged by them. Learning to recognize these experiences as they arise and knowing they are simply part of the experience of meditation can be helpful. It's not just you!

These challenges will most certainly arise for anyone practicing meditation, including you. When we recognize them, they become less of a barrier or "problem." We can learn to observe them with curiosity and nonjudgment.

1. AVERSION

This is the experience of "not wanting" or "not liking." Any time we experience something and have the reaction of dislike, or the desire to make that experience go away, it could be described as aversion. This might include feelings of fear, anger, irritation, disgust, or resentment.

2. CRAVING OR WANTING

This can be as subtle as wanting to feel a little more relaxed and peaceful, or as strong as an intense urge or craving.

3. RESTLESSNESS OR AGITATION

This can be experienced physically, as in an itchy discomfort or strong desire to move during meditation, or can be experienced as the mind feeling restless or uncomfortable.

4. DROWSINESS OR SLEEPINESS

This could be physical sleepiness or just mental sluggishness. It might be in the mind, the body, or both.

5. DOUBT

Doubt might be experienced as a sense of doubt about yourself ("I can't do this practice"), or doubt about the practice and its utility ("This is ridiculous. Why would people just sit there and watch their breath?"). Doubt can especially tricky because it is often very convincing.

It may help to remember that the type of meditation we are practicing has been around for thousands of years and has helped millions of people transform their lives. There is no one who cannot participate in meditation; it is accessible to anyone who wishes to practice. It can also be a challenging practice. The important part is to stay with it, and when these challenges arise (which they will) to bring them, too, into your awareness.

Noticing Triggers Worksheet
HANDOUT 2.2

Pay attention this week to what triggers you or to times when you feel reactive. Use the following questions to bring awareness to the details of the experience as it is happening.

Day/ date	Situation/trigger	What sensations did you experience?	What moods, feelings, or emotions?	What were your thoughts?	What did you do?
Example: Friday 3/26	An argument with a friend.	Tightness in chest, cold, clammy palms, heart beating fast.	Anxiety, craving.	I really need something to get me through this.	Took a walk, later talked with friend about what upset me.

A New Relationship with Discomfort
HANDOUT 2.3

THEME

Most of us tend to either give in to craving or fight hard to resist it. This session focuses on learning to experience triggers and cravings differently. We begin by learning to identify what triggers us, then observing how these triggers lead to all the sensations, thoughts, and emotions that are often part of craving. We practice observing the experience without "automatically" reacting. Mindfulness can help bring this process into our awareness, allowing us to disrupt the "automatic" chain of reactions that often follows a trigger and giving us greater freedom to make choices that in the long run make us happier.

INTEGRATING PRACTICE INTO YOUR WEEK

1. As best you can, practice the body scan daily this week and note your experiences on the Daily Practice Tracking Sheet.

2. Fill out the Noticing Triggers Worksheet each day, noting the thoughts, urges or cravings, emotions (e.g., angry, sad, anxious, happy), and body sensations (e.g., tight in the chest, jittery) you experience. If no triggers or thoughts of using come up on a particular day, you can simply make a note of that. You could also note other types of triggers, for example, things that bring up anger, shame, or any behaviors you would like to change.

3. Continue with the mindfulness of a daily activity practice. You can use the same activity or choose a different one. Bring your full attention to that activity, noticing the sensations, sights, sounds, thoughts, and even emotions that arise.

Daily Practice Tracking Sheet

HANDOUT 2.4

Instructions: Each day, record your mindfulness practice, also noting any barriers, observations, or comments.

Day/date	Formal practice with audio recording: How long?	Mindfulness of daily activities	Observations, comments, or challenges (aversion, craving, sleepiness, restlessness, doubt)
	____ minutes	What activities?	
	____ minutes	What activities?	
	____ minutes	What activities?	
	____ minutes	What activities?	
	____ minutes	What activities?	
	____ minutes	What activities?	

From Reacting to Responding

> Between stimulus and response, there is a space.
> In that space is our power to choose our response.
> In our response lies our growth and our freedom.
>   —VIKTOR E. FRANKL

Materials

- Bell
- Whiteboard/markers
- Handout 3.1: SOBER Space
- Handout 3.2: Session 3 Theme and Daily Practice: From Reacting to Responding
- Handout 3.3: Daily Practice Tracking Sheet
- Audio Files: Sitting Meditation (Breath), SOBER Space

Theme

Practicing mindfulness can increase our awareness and help us make more skillful choices in our daily lives. Because breathing is always here for us, pausing and paying attention to the feeling of the breath is a way to return to the present and bring awareness back to the body. With this presence and awareness, we are often less reactive and can make decisions from a steadier, clearer place that is more aligned with how we want to be in the world. The "SOBER space" is a practice that can help us integrate skills from the formal sitting or body scan meditations into situations and challenges we encounter in our daily lives.

Goals

- Introduce breath meditation.
- Introduce SOBER space.
- Continue practices and discussion of integrating mindfulness into everyday living.

Session Outline

- Check-In
- Awareness of Hearing (Practice 3.1)
- Practice Review
- Breath Meditation (Practice 3.2) and Review
- False Refuge (Practice 3.3)
- SOBER Space (Practice 3.4)
- Daily Practice
- Closing

Practice for This Week

- Breath Meditation
- SOBER Space

CHECK-IN

The check-in is intended to bring attention to a present-moment experience (i.e., "Describe one or two things you notice right now, such as sensations, emotions, or thoughts") or to get in touch with a value or intention (i.e., "What is most important to you to focus on in today's session?" or "What are your intentions for today?"). Facilitators can make use of either or both of these practices at the beginning of each session.

AWARENESS OF HEARING

Mindfulness is of limited benefit if confined to just the cushion. Although "formal" practices are crucial to building a strong foundation, the real practice, at least in this program, is the translation and integration of these perspectives and skills to day-to-day living. This is first introduced with the "mindfulness of a daily activity" exercise in Session 1, and is further emphasized in the current session. Beginning with the awareness of hearing exercise (Practice 3.1), this session focuses on simple ways to bring attention to activities in which we are constantly engaged but often carry out without much awareness. These activities are so automatic for most of us that bringing attention to the actual experience, such as hearing, can be quite new and interesting.

This brief meditation has an intention similar to the body scan (i.e., bringing attention to what is already occurring) and to all others in this program. We are exploring our experiences through the different senses (i.e., seeing, hearing, smelling, tasting, physical sensation, and consciousness of these experiences).

In inquiry following the hearing exercise, and following the seeing exercise described in Session 4, we revisit the idea of automatic pilot, returning to the initial intention of stepping out of default or automatic mode and observing what happens when attention and awareness are brought to any activity, no matter how mundane or routine it might seem. These exercises often illuminate just how automatic the processes of seeing and hearing are, how our minds repeatedly label and categorize these experiences, and how this can obstruct our true vision or direct contact with raw experience. We have found the seeing/hearing exercises are useful ways to practice direct observation and to begin noticing the mind's tendency to immediately jump in to assess, label, categorize, and judge.

FACILITATOR: What did people notice in the awareness of hearing exercise?

PARTICIPANT 1: I heard something moving on that side of the room and thought, "What is that?" Then I really wanted to open my eyes.

FACILITATOR: So you noticed several things—hearing a sound, noticing it was from that side of the room, the thought "What is that noise?," and an urge to open your eyes. Anything else?

PARTICIPANT 1: Yeah, I felt like it was cheating.

FACILITATOR: So another thought, "I'm cheating." Was there any judgment?

PARTICIPANT 1: Maybe a little bit, like "I shouldn't need to break the rules."

PARTICIPANT 2: I noticed the pattern of the noise of the traffic outside as the traffic lights changed. I started thinking about how the cars were stopping at the red light, because of how it would suddenly get quiet. Then there must have been a green light, because the traffic sounds started again.

FACILITATOR: Okay, you noticed sounds and the pattern of those sounds, and maybe the mind labeling this as "cars" or "traffic"? Then some thoughts about why the pattern was like that. It sounds like the mind began explaining and maybe even picturing the scene that the pattern was related to.

PARTICIPANT 2: Yeah. At first it was just sound, and then I noticed this pattern, and then there was a thought about what was happening out there.

FACILITATOR: The mind wanting to make sense of what you were hearing. So is this similar to or different from how you typically experience sound throughout your day?

PARTICIPANT 2: Pretty different. Normally I don't really notice particular sounds, unless it's my name or something annoying, or a song I like or something.

FACILITATOR: This simple practice is something you can try pretty much anywhere, anytime. You can close your eyes or not, depending on the situation, and just listen to the sounds around you, to the textures and patterns. Thoughts will arise about what you're hearing, the attention will wander. Just notice that, and see if you can come back to simply hearing sounds as sound, noticing the texture, the loudness, the softness, the pattern of it.

DAILY PRACTICE REVIEW

After 2 weeks of practicing the body scan meditation on their own, participants may have a wider variety of responses and experiences. The body scan practice is intended to help clients raise awareness of physical sensation in the present moment. It is a way to practice paying attention to the body's states and responses from a nonattached, observer's perspective. It may also foster awareness of habits of the mind and barriers to practice. It can be helpful to revisit the Common Challenges in Meditation Practice (and in Daily Life) handout (Handout 2.1) as examples of aversion, craving, restlessness, sleepiness, or doubt arise.

FACILITATOR: What were people's experiences with the body scan practice this week?

PARTICIPANT 1: It was a lot easier this time.

FACILITATOR: When you say "easier," what did you notice that was different?

PARTICIPANT 1: I did better. I could stay more focused, and could get through the whole thing.

FACILITATOR: So you noticed that you were more able to focus, maybe your mind stayed with the body more and wandered to other thoughts less.

PARTICIPANT 1: Yeah.

FACILITATOR: And it sounds, too, like there's a judgment with that, that this is "good" or "better." Do you remember any thoughts that occurred while you were doing the body scan, about how you were doing?

PARTICIPANT 1: Yeah. (*Laughs.*) I had thoughts like, "Oh, cool, I'm getting better at this."

FACILITATOR: So you're having this experience, a more direct experience, of the body, the sensations, etcetera. Then a thought comes, evaluating this experience.

PARTICIPANT 1: Yeah. That's what I did.

FACILITATOR: There's nothing wrong here; we're just noticing whatever is happening. Getting to know our minds. Other experiences? Tell me about integrating practice into your life this past week.

PARTICIPANT 2: I tried to do the body scan. I would keep starting, then would turn off the recording. I just couldn't do it.

FACILITATOR: Interesting. So what happened? When you say you'd get started and then you'd stop, what happened when you felt like you needed to stop? What do you remember about that?

PARTICIPANT 2: Um, I . . . I don't know. Like last night, I just wasn't calm enough to sit through it. My mind was scattered, and I wasn't able to really get into it.

FACILITATOR: Okay, this is a really common experience so I'm glad you brought it up. Do you remember the common challenges we talked about last week? Which one might this be?

PARTICIPANT 2: Right—restlessness. I definitely felt that one. Maybe aversion, too.

FACILITATOR: Great. I encourage you to keep noticing this. What does your body feel like? What thoughts are happening? Maybe there's some emotion there, too. Maybe irritation, shame, maybe even anger. So let's see what comes up this week.

It sounds like, from what you just said, there might be an assumption that the mind needs to be calm, not scattered, to be able to do this practice. This also comes up a lot. What would happen if you tried staying with it when the mind felt scattered and just noticed what happened?

We set this time aside to practice, and then something gets in the way, either an external distraction like the phone or the kids or something internal like your mind going in 18 different directions, and it's really easy to get frustrated and discouraged. This is something we'll continue to talk about in upcoming weeks, because it will continue to happen. The important part is bringing awareness to what's happening during the practice and in the rest of our lives. So it's okay if distractions happen. Recognize that you are distracted, and maybe just check out what *that* feels like. What is my mind doing? What does this feel like in my body? It's another opportunity to pay attention, to observe our experience.

Often in this third week, further barriers and frustrations arise. There is ongoing doubt about doing the practice "right," and questions may begin to arise about its purpose.

PARTICIPANT: I'm practicing what you are trying to teach us. This is a new thing, and I want to get as much out of it as possible. So I was thinking the other day, how do you incorporate this into . . . I guess I'm not getting it as far as where all this leads to make it something that you would do that would help with urges . . .

FACILITATOR: Yes, okay. And this is actually the focus of today's session. How can this foundation that you're building with all of the practices we're doing help you in daily situations that really matter? So how might the body scan be used or be useful with urges, cravings, recovery? Do people have ideas? [Here the facilitator is eliciting ideas and experiences from the group rather than immediately trying to provide an answer.]

PARTICIPANT: Well, like with the worksheet you gave us last week, I realized I was only putting down emotions, and so I started trying to notice the physical reactions I was having, too. I can see how doing the body scan every day has helped me do that. I don't think I would notice those physical reactions in my body. It's almost like sometimes I don't even have a body. So practicing noticing helps me actually feel what's happening in my body.

FACILITATOR: Okay, yes. And how might that help with urges or cravings? Or any other behaviors in your life?

PARTICIPANT: If you can feel where it's coming from in the body you can focus on that part and just relax it a little bit. Slowing down and noticing and taking stock of what's going on instead of just reaching for a drink or reacting.

A primary focus of this session is to prepare participants to move into working with high-risk situations by closely observing the reactions that often feel overwhelming and instantaneous. The Noticing Triggers Worksheet (Handout 2.2), assigned in the previous session and part of this week's daily practice discussion, is designed to bring the same curiosity to thoughts and emotions that we have been bringing to physical sensations. By bringing attention to what is happening, via any of the senses, we can then begin to observe the associated feelings and reactions that arise around these initial experiences. In discussing the worksheet, we again practice discerning thought, emotion, and physical sensation.

The final column of the Noticing Triggers Worksheet assesses behavior. The purpose of this component is not to evaluate or change the behavior but to begin to expand awareness to include behavioral responses and their consequences. Typically, we do not place a great deal of emphasis on this facet. Sometimes we simply ask, "So you felt angry and hurt, your heart was racing, and you noticed some thoughts about how you couldn't go through this again. How did you respond to this experience? What did you do?"

We have found that discussion of the Noticing Triggers Worksheet often provokes storytelling. To continue to maintain a focus on direct experience, we gently redirect participants to the experience rather than the story of the preceding incident. This can be done by explicitly stating that for this exercise we are only interested in participants' direct experiences and their reactions, keeping the description of the trigger to a few words if possible (it is sometimes helpful to ask participants to just read what they wrote on the sheet). Facilitators may need to redirect several times in a session, especially in these beginning weeks.

FACILITATOR: For the discussion about this exercise, I am interested in your reactions and responses more than in the situation that triggered them. Part of what we're doing in here is taking the focus off of that other person, the situation, or the story, and bringing attention to ourselves—to our body, mind, and heart, and how this whole internal system here is responding. So something happened, whatever it was, that triggered you. Tell me, what was the first thing you noticed about your own reaction? Was it physical? A thought? An urge?

PARTICIPANT: I had this experience 3 days ago. I ride the bus a lot and see different areas where people are still using. It takes me to this feeling of being really grateful. And the feeling in my body is like, "Oh, thank God I am not there anymore." At the same time I feel bad for these people.

FACILITATOR: Okay, did you write about this one? Would you be willing to read what you wrote there on your worksheet?

PARTICIPANT: I wrote, "Event: seeing people using on the street. Sensation in body: lonely, sad."

FACILITATOR: So there's emotion—sadness, loneliness. And a memory of yourself out there in the past.

There was an image of yourself out there and some relief that that time is over. You had the thought "Thank God that's not me out there."

Then you mentioned, too, feeling sadness and loneliness. Did you notice any physical sensation when you felt that sadness and loneliness?

PARTICIPANT: Just a feeling that I don't ever want that to happen again.

FACILITATOR: So there's a thought about never wanting to be out there again. How about physical sensations? Anything you noticed?

PARTICIPANT: Yeah, tightness in my stomach.

FACILITATOR: It seems like a lot of thoughts about not wanting to be out there, and some memories, maybe, and a lot of emotion—the sadness and loneliness and relief and tightness in your stomach. This is great, that you are noticing all of this.

As in this example, often clients have difficulty discerning a thought from an emotion. In future sessions, we might bring more focus to responses to these initial experiences, such as judgments or frustration for feeling a certain way. In this session, however, the primary focus is on noticing and differentiating between the different components of these initial reactions.

BREATH MEDITATION AND REVIEW

This session introduces participants to formal sitting practice (Practice 3.2: breath meditation). Encouraging and coaching participants to find a posture that supports a relaxed alertness and a sense of self-respect and dignity can support these qualities in the mind. Stiffness can bring about harshness, while laxity can foster sleepiness or fogginess. At this point, many participants still have perceptions of meditation as a "trancelike" state or as a relaxation exercise. We continue to emphasize that these practices are about waking up to our present experience and increasing our awareness, not floating away or escaping. We are practicing staying in this moment rather than habitually calling up the past or inventing a future. Posture can support this intention.

Inquiry following this first breath meditation offers an opportunity for facilitators to again emphasize the intent of this practice; simply observing our experience. It is unrealistic to expect that the mind will not wander when our minds have been "practicing" wandering our entire lives. Beginning inquiry with a question such as "What did people notice about their minds as they did this exercise?" can encourage discussion of what actually happened rather than what participants believe they were supposed to experience. Bringing some humor and levity here can be helpful; it can be difficult, even for us facilitators, to keep the mind on a single focus even for just one breath!

Because beginning a practice can be so challenging, length of sitting meditations, especially in these beginning weeks, has been the topic of interesting discussions among facilitators of mindfulness-based groups. Colleagues and teachers of related programs have begun the course with brief meditations, lasting perhaps 10 minutes, and likewise suggest 10 minutes of sitting for daily practice. Some stay with that period throughout the course, while others describe slowly increasing the time over the 8 weeks to 20–30 minutes. The longer in-session practices allow clients to encounter, and possibly move through, experiences of physical and affective discomfort. Many participants become more restless after about 15 minutes, and encouraging them to stay with this experience rather than stopping at the peak of their uneasiness allows them to observe this discomfort, refrain from reacting in habitual ways, and learn new responses.

We have found that many participants will listen to the whole recording during the first week and continue to do so throughout the course, and even beyond the course's end, while others struggle to practice at all. The best approach to length of practice continues to be an interesting issue, worthy of further discussion and exploration. We recommend that facilitators follow their own instincts, while being careful not to underestimate or shortchange their participants' willingness or ability.

FALSE REFUGE EXERCISE

This exercise invites participants to reflect on what they are actually seeking or longing for when turning toward substance use or another addictive behavior. These needs and desires are then listed on the board and often include a longing for relief, freedom, connection, or nurturing or a desire to feel seen and valued. Seeing these listed on the board not only highlights the shared human experience of some of these longings, it also helps to depathologize the craving that often masks them. Participants are then asked what they actually end up getting as a result of engaging in the behavior, and this is listed in a second column, next to the first. This list often includes shame, regret, damaged relationships, loss of self-respect, loss of trust, and financial stress, among other things. The discussion following the exercise invites recognition of the humanity and wholesome aspects of these longings, along with the failure of the behavior to truly deliver on its promise of meeting these needs, although it may appear to do so in the short term.

SOBER SPACE

The formal meditation practices taught in this course are intended to provide the foundation for integrating new perspectives and behaviors into daily life. The

SOBER (*S*top, *O*bserve, *B*reath, *E*xpand, *R*espond) space (Practice 3.3 and Handout 3.1) is an adaptation of the 3-minute breathing space used in MBCT. Although we have found the SOBER space to be one of the most useful daily life practices, it is not introduced until Session 3 because of the importance of establishing a foundation to support it. By Session 3, participants have been introduced to the idea of stopping and stepping out of autopilot by shifting attention to direct experience. They have now had 2 weeks of observing the physical sensations in their bodies, laying the groundwork for the "observe" step. Similarly, bringing focus to the breath now has a context, and participants have had some familiarity with this practice as well. In a high-risk or stressful situation, experience with meditation can help individuals draw upon these practices. We continue to practice the SOBER space in future sessions, presenting it slightly differently each time to continue to generalize the skills.

As in MBCT, we often describe it using the image of an hourglass: we begin with a broad focus, then narrow the focus to the breath, and finally expand back out to a wider awareness, illustrating the hourglass, alongside the SOBER acronym, on the whiteboard. We also describe it as shifting the spotlight of awareness from the outer situation to the inner experience (i.e., sensations, thoughts, and emotions) and then back out again.

As with many of the practices, there are often expectations for a certain outcome or result. Participants will often comment that it "worked" or "didn't work." Similar to the body scan, sitting meditation, and urge surfing, we emphasize that the purpose of the practice is to step out of autopilot and observe; it is to practice noticing, not necessarily to feel differently or to change anything. We often ask what participants noticed, and if there were differences in their experiences during the initial observation and what they noticed when expanding awareness again to the body and mind following the breath focus. It is important to do this carefully, so as not to imply that there *should* be a difference, perhaps even commenting that sometimes there will be and sometimes there won't be, and the important piece is to bring attention to *whatever* is happening.

DAILY PRACTICE

In these first several weeks, we encourage participants to spend some time with each of the meditation exercises introduced. Experiencing these different forms of meditation allows a deeper experience of the practice and offers a variety from which participants may choose as they begin to form their individual programs of practice in the final weeks and beyond. Following Session 3, we suggest that participants practice with the breath and other sitting meditation audio recordings as many days as possible during the upcoming week (Handout 3.2). We encourage them to stay with the sitting meditation for the week rather than returning to the body scan and reiterate that mindfulness includes observation of reactions to the practice (e.g., preference of one over another, resistance or restlessness, or doubt about the practice "working"). We also emphasize that, as with any new skill, the beginning can be frustrating, and it often takes time and effort to learn something new.

The second part of the home practice is to begin integrating the SOBER space into daily life (Handout 3.1), both during routine daily activities and in higher-stress situations. Integrating this daily may sound overwhelming, as most of us have been practicing "unawareness" throughout much of our lives. However, by regularly practicing this technique, we begin integrating it into daily life, replacing the often deeply ingrained habit of reactivity with a more mindful response of stopping and observing. We are retraining the mind, and new habits require repetition. If the group seems to be having difficulty integrating practice into daily life, facilitators can ask for ideas or creative ways of remembering to use these tools (e.g., while waiting at the bus stop, when getting annoyed with a spouse, or right before eating a meal). Participants are also asked to complete the Daily Practice Tracking Sheet (Handout 3.3).

CLOSING

As in previous sessions, it is helpful to mark the end of the session with a few moments of silence, followed by the sound of a bell, and a brief one- to two-word description of what participants are noticing about their thoughts, feelings, or sensations in the moment.

Awareness of Hearing
PRACTICE 3.1

Intentions

+ Bringing awareness to sensory experience versus content

+ Noticing the mind's tendency to immediately jump in to assess, label, categorize, and judge, and how this can obstruct our true vision or raw experience

+ Attention to hearing as a practice to help "get out of our heads"

Take a moment to settle into your chair or cushion. You can close your eyes or leave them open, however you feel most comfortable. Allowing yourself to arrive here in the room, feeling your body in the chair or on the cushion, the sensations of your breath as it enters and leaves the body. Now just letting your attention rest on the experience of hearing, noticing sounds. Hearing sounds inside the room and outside it. Hearing sounds both inside and outside of your body. Maybe listening for the quietest sound. As best you can, letting go of ideas or stories about the sounds and just hearing them as patterns, loud or soft, high pitched or low pitched. Hearing the texture of the sounds. You don't need to try to hear anything in particular, just allowing the sounds to come to you, as though you are listening with your whole body, with all of your senses, open and receptive to the experience of sound.

There is no need to analyze or think about the sounds . . . as best you can, just experiencing them. If you find that you are having thoughts such as "This is weird" or "I don't want to do this" or "I'm not doing this right," simply notice that as well, and gently bring your attention back to the direct experience of hearing.

Whenever you become aware that your attention has wandered off, or you have started to *think* about what is being heard rather than simply experiencing it, gently bring your attention back to simply hearing.

Based on Segal, Williams, and Teasdale (2013).

Intentions

+ Practicing *repeatedly returning* focus to a present-centered experience (breath)

+ Noticing the tendency of the mind to wander and get caught in thoughts and stories, and practicing nonjudgmental awareness

+ Disabusing ideas about meditation being a "trancelike" state, or simply a relaxation exercise

---

Take a moment to settle into a natural, relaxed, and alert posture, with your feet flat on the floor if you are in a chair. It may be helpful to sit away from the back of the chair so that your spine is self-supporting. We pay attention to how we sit during meditation because it can affect our experience. We want a relaxed posture, with our spine and shoulders relaxed. The head can be tilted a little forward so the eyes, if open, look down at the floor. Find a posture that embodies dignity and self-sufficiency while still remaining relaxed, not stiff. So take a moment now to find that posture for yourself, that sense of relaxed alertness.

You may keep your eyes open or closed, whichever feels comfortable to you. Throughout the course, you might want to experiment with both keeping your eyes open and allowing them to close for these exercises. Sometimes it is helpful to start with eyes closed to better focus your attention on your experience of what's going on in your mind and body, but please do what is most comfortable for you. If you keep your eyes open, let your gaze fall on a spot a few feet in front of you on the floor or on the wall, keeping your focus soft so you are just letting your eyes rest there, not really looking *at* anything.

Now allowing your belly to soften so the breath can flow easily in and out. Softening the muscles in the face, the jaw, the shoulders, and neck.

Letting go as best you can of whatever thoughts or ideas you might have come in with today. Take an intention deep breath if that helps you settle. And just allowing the past to fall away, and letting go of thinking or worrying about what comes next. Seeing if you can allow yourself for the next little while to just be right here. There's nothing else you need to be doing right now. You might begin by bringing your attention to physical sensations. Bringing awareness to physical sensation can be a helpful way to come into the present, because no matter where the mind is, the body is always present. So maybe now just feeling the weight of your body in the chair or on your cushion. Noticing the places where your body makes contact with the floor and with your chair or cushion. See if you can feel even the light pressure of your clothing against your skin or maybe the air touching your hands or your face.

Now gathering your attention and bringing it to the very next breath. You might feel this in your abdomen as it rises and falls with the inhale and exhale. If it is helpful in focusing your attention, you can put your hand on your belly to help feel the rising and falling. Or you might choose to focus on the area right beneath your nostrils, feeling the air as it enters and leaves the body.

Choose the area where you feel the sensations most strongly and, as best you can, keep your attention there, feeling these sensations of breathing. Maybe beginning with just one inhale—seeing if you can keep your attention on the sensation of breath from

(continued)

the beginning of one inhale to when it turns around and becomes an exhale. Then let go and try it again. Follow with your awareness the physical sensations and how they change with each inbreath and outbreath. Seeing if you can notice the slight pauses between the inbreath and the outbreath, and then again the slight pause before the next inbreath.

We are not trying to change the breathing in any way—let your body breathe the way it naturally does. We're simply observing the sensations as it breathes, allowing your experience to be just as it is, without judging or needing to change it.

As we sit here with our focus on the sensations of breath, the attention will inevitably wander off to something else. It might have already happened. This is natural; it is simply what our minds are in the habit of doing. When you become aware that your attention has gotten caught up in thoughts or stories, simply notice that. You might even gently say to yourself "Not now" and allow your mind to release the thought, bringing attention once again to the very next breath. There is no need to judge yourself when the mind wanders, because it inevitably will. Simply notice, let go, and begin again with the next breath. This noticing and beginning again is part of the practice.

This may happen a hundred times, and that is okay. Simply guide your attention back to the breath, beginning again.

Whenever you find yourself "carried away" from awareness in the moment by thoughts or the intensity of physical sensations, as best you can, bring a gentle, caring curiosity to your experience. Then reconnect with the here and now by bringing your awareness back to the sensations of the breath.

In these last few moments, renewing your intention to stay present, as best you can, beginning again and again, as many times as you need to. Letting go of the thoughts and arriving again right here, with attention on the sensations of breathing.

Now gently expanding your focus to include the room around you and the people here. When you are ready, slowly and gently allow your eyes to open, staying with this sense of awareness.

Intentions

+ Recognizing needs that often underlie craving

+ Exploring whether addictive behavior truly fulfills these underlying needs

+ Recognizing addictive behavior as an ineffective way of getting our needs met

---

I'd like to invite you to take a moment to reflect on the behavior that brought you here, whether it is substance use or another behavior that doesn't serve you. You may even close your eyes for a moment, if that is comfortable for you, and consider the moments or situations in which you are most tempted to engage in this behavior, or experience a strong craving to engage in the behavior. Considering what these situations are for you.

Now, seeing if you might turn the lens from the behavior to what is happening for you in these moments, asking yourself what it is you are actually, mostly deeply longing for. What need do you hope the substance or behavior will fill?

As you are ready, you can open your eyes if they are closed.

1. What needs came up for you in that reflection? [List in one column on the board and highlight any common themes.]

2. Okay, after engaging in this behavior, what do you actually end up getting? Maybe it's what you were wanting, or maybe not. [List in a second column on the board and illustrate common themes.]

3. Any reactions as you look at this? [Elicit from the group.]

What I am struck by here is how wholesome these needs/desires are. Of course we want these things. We are just trying to take care of ourselves, to be happy. Nothing wrong with that. So what's the problem? [Elicit responses from the group.]

Intentions

✦ Integrating mindfulness into daily life by practicing the shift out of "autopilot" and into awareness, especially in situations in which we tend to be reactive

✦ Establishing a clear, focused, and portable practice for higher-stress situations

✦ Observing whatever is arising, not necessarily changing our experience or "feeling better"—which may allow for choice in the face of challenging situations

---

We have been doing a lot of longer meditations, both here and at home. We now want to begin to bring this practice into our lives in a way that can help us cope with daily challenges, stressful situations, triggers, and so forth. So this is an exercise you can do almost anywhere, anytime, because it is very brief and quite simple. This is an especially useful exercise when we find ourselves in a stressful or high-risk situation. As we discussed last week, often when we are triggered by things in ourselves or in our environment, we tend to go into automatic pilot, which can result in our behaving in ways that are not in our best interest. This is a technique that can be used to help us step out of that automatic mode and become more aware and mindful of our actions.

1. The first step is to **stop** or **slow down** right where you are, and make the choice to **shift** out of automatic pilot by bringing awareness to your experience in this moment.

2. Now just **observe** what is happening in this moment, in your body, thoughts, and emotions.

3. Then gather your attention and focus just on the sensations of **breathing.**

4. **Expand** awareness to check in again on your sense of the whole body, and the thoughts and emotions that you notice. They may be the same as before, or maybe they have changed.

5. Now, notice that whatever you are experiencing in your body, mind, or emotions, you can have a choice in how you **respond.** We'll talk about this final step a bit more next time.

Let's try this now. You may either close your eyes or keep them open.

1. The first step is to stop, shifting out of automatic mode.

2. The next step is to observe what is happening in your mind and body right now. What is your experience in this moment? What sensations do you notice? Is there any discomfort or tension in your body? What thoughts are present? What emotion might you notice, and where is that in your body? Just acknowledging that this is your experience right now.

3. So now you have a sense of what is going on right now in this moment. Now gathering your attention, focusing attention on sensations of the breath, just for a few breaths, as best you can.

(continued)

4. And the next step is to allow your awareness to expand, and include a sense of your entire body, and any thoughts you are having, and any emotions. Holding it all in this softer, more spacious awareness.

5. Sensing that this is a place from which you might be able to respond to any situation with more awareness.

And then, when you are ready, gently allowing your eyes to open.

Adapted from Segal, Williams, and Teasdale (2013). Copyright © 2013 The Guilford Press. Used by permission.

SOBER Space
HANDOUT 3.1

This is an exercise that you can do almost anywhere, anytime, because it is brief and quite simple. It can be used in the midst of a high-risk or stressful situation, if you are upset about something, or when you are experiencing urges and cravings to use. It can help you step out of automatic pilot, becoming less reactive and more aware and mindful in your response.

A way to help remember these steps is the acronym SOBER.

S—Stop (or Shift). When you are in a stressful or risky situation, or even just at random times throughout the day, remember to stop or slow down and shift your attention from the situation to what is happening in your experience. This is the first step in stepping out of automatic pilot.

O—Observe. Observe the sensations that are happening in your body. Also observe any emotions, moods, or thoughts you are having. Just notice as much as you can about your experience.

B—Breath. Gather your attention and bring it to the sensations of your breath.

E—Expand. Expand your awareness to again include the rest of your body, your mind, and your emotions, seeing if you can gently hold it all in awareness.

R—Respond. Respond mindfully (vs. react), with awareness of what is truly needed in the situation and how you can best take care of yourself. Whatever is happening in your mind and body, you still have a choice in how you respond.

From Reacting to Responding
HANDOUT 3.2

THEME

Mindfulness practices can help us increase awareness and subsequently make more skillful choices in our everyday lives. Because breathing is always a present-moment experience, pausing and paying attention to sensations of the breath can be a way to return to the present moment and come back into the body. When we are more present, we are often more aware and less reactive and can make decisions from a stronger, clearer place. The SOBER space is a practice that can extend this quality of mindfulness from formal sitting or lying-down practice into the daily situations and challenges we encounter.

INTEGRATING PRACTICE INTO YOUR WEEK

1. Practice with the sitting meditation audio recordings this week and note your experiences on the Daily Practice Tracking Sheet.

2. Begin integrating the SOBER space into your daily life. It is best to practice this in both day-to-day situations as well as in challenging situations. Make a note of your practice on the Daily Practice Tracking Sheet.

Daily Practice Tracking Sheet
HANDOUT 3.3

Instructions: Each day, record your mindfulness practice, also noting any barriers, observations, or comments.

Day/ date	Formal practice with audio files: How long?	SOBER space	Notes/comments
	_____ minutes	How often? In what situations?	
	_____ minutes	How often? In what situations?	
	_____ minutes	How often? In what situations?	
	_____ minutes	How often? In what situations?	
	_____ minutes	How often? In what situations?	
	_____ minutes	How often? In what situations?	
	_____ minutes	How often? In what situations?	

Mindfulness in Challenging Situations

When we scratch the wound and give in to our addictions, we do not allow the wound to heal. But when we instead experience the raw quality of the itch or pain of the wound and do not scratch it, we actually allow the wound to heal. So not giving in to our addictions is about healing at a very basic level.

It is about truly nourishing ourselves.

—PEMA CHÖDRÖN

Materials

- Bell
- Whiteboard/markers
- Handout 4.1: Session 4 Theme and Daily Practice: Mindfulness in Challenging Situations
- Handout 4.2: Daily Practice Tracking Sheet
- Audio File: Sitting Meditation (Sound, Breath, Sensation, Thought, Emotion)

Theme

In this session, we focus on staying present in challenging situations that have previously been associated with substance use or other reactive behaviors. We learn how to relate differently to cravings or urges to use substances and practice responding to highly evocative stimuli with awareness rather than reacting automatically or out of habit.

Goals

- Increase awareness of individual challenging situations and of the sensations, emotions, and thoughts that tend to arise.

- Practice staying with intense or uncomfortable sensations or emotions rather than avoiding or attempting to get rid of them.

- Learn skills to help stay present and not automatically give in to pressure to use substances in situations that have previously been associated with use.

- Introduce mindful walking as another practice in awareness of various physical sensations and in bringing mindful attention into daily life.

Session Outline

- Check-In
- Awareness of Seeing (Practice 4.1)
- Practice Review
- Sitting Meditation: Sound, Breath, Sensation, Thought (Practice 4.2)
- Individual and Common Relapse Risks
- SOBER Space in a Challenging Situation (Practice 4.3)
- Walking Meditation (Practice 4.4)
- Daily Practice
- Closing

Practice for This Week

- Sitting Meditation
- Walking Meditation or Mindful Walking
- SOBER Space

CHECK-IN

Consistent with previous weeks, this session begins with a brief one- to two-word check-in. Participants are invited to keep these descriptions focused on present-moment experience and to notice the tendency of the mind to anticipate and prepare a response while they are awaiting their turn. Facilitators might encourage the group to try *not* preplanning, to listen fully to the others in the group, and notice what arises when their turn comes.

AWARENESS OF SEEING

In the previous session, we introduced exercises to help bring mindfulness from the formal meditations into daily life. This fourth session is designed to continue this integration, with a specific focus on bringing mindfulness into more challenging areas or situations that tend to elicit reactive behavior. Experiential exercises focus on using some of the familiar practices and skills, such as the SOBER space, in the context of a challenging situation. The session begins with a brief exercise in mindful seeing (Practice 4.1). If there is an opportunity to look outside, guidance might include observing the wind moving through the trees or people or cars passing by. In the absence of a window, suggestions might include noticing light and shadow, texture, or color or shapes in the room, while also noticing deeply habitual ways in which the mind works (i.e., automatically labeling and categorizing what is seen).

DAILY PRACTICE REVIEW

In reviewing experiences with the sitting meditation and SOBER space, it is once again helpful to dispel any expectations for a specific outcome. Participants often have continued beliefs about relaxation or calmness as indicative of a "successful" meditation. Reminding the group that the intention of these practices is to become aware of the tendencies of the mind is often necessary, even in this fourth week. In reviewing the sitting meditation, we continue to highlight that observing a wandering or restless mind is part of the practice and an opportunity to observe our reactions to these tendencies.

SITTING MEDITATION: SOUND, BREATH, SENSATION, THOUGHT

The first sitting practice, introduced in the previous session (Practice 3.2), began with a basic awareness of sensations of the breath. Each of the following sessions builds upon this practice, expanding the field of awareness to include other sense experiences. The current session's beginning meditation (Practice 4.2) begins again with awareness of sound, shifts to awareness of breath, then to sensations and thoughts. Future sessions will continue to work with these experiences as well as introduce mindfulness of emotion.

Participants have now worked with the sitting (breath) practice for a week and are likely running into both familiar and new challenges.

PARTICIPANT: The long pauses in the recording drove me crazy.

FACILITATOR: Okay—what did you notice? What was coming up for you during the pauses?

PARTICIPANT: Oh man, I was getting really agitated.

FACILITATOR: Were you noticing that agitation or restlessness at the time?

PARTICIPANT: Oh, yeah. I knew I was agitated.

FACILITATOR: Great. What happened next?

PARTICIPANT: I'd notice it, try to just sort of let it go, or let it be, then try going back to noticing my breathing. I was trying to just sit with it and let the agitation be there but come back into the moment. Sometimes my mind would immediately go to watching the clock, then the thought "When is this going to end?"

FACILITATOR: So you were noticing agitation, while also keeping some aware-ness on your breath—trying to stay present with that? Then thoughts about the clock, the time, and when this would end. Were there sensations you noticed?

PARTICIPANT: Yeah, my body felt sort of itchy all over, and I just wanted to move.

FACILITATOR: Great. You're noticing agitation, how that feels in the body, then watching how the mind is reacting. I'm curious—is that feeling of wanting to move or escape familiar?

Often by this point in the course, clients begin to notice changes in their prac-tice and in their responses to what they are experiencing.

PARTICIPANT 1: Early on, I was drifting in and out more noticeably, distracted and hearing other things, but last night, I found my thoughts were pretty much focused on just my breathing, so that was kind of pleasurable.

FACILITATOR: So you're noticing that your mind is able to remain a little more focused. Was your mind not wandering as much, or were you able to notice the wandering sooner?

PARTICIPANT 1: Kind of both. It was wandering less, and it was easier when I did notice to rein it in.

FACILITATOR: And you said it was pleasurable to have that increased focus. What did you notice about that pleasure? What did it feel like?

PARTICIPANT 1: Kind of a relaxation and relief. It feels like it alleviates stress, physical tension.

PARTICIPANT 2: Me too. It feels like it's getting easier each time to stay focused on the exercise. I'm still wandering a bit, but I catch myself starting to fade away, then come back. I just started getting an itch when you said to bring awareness to any place of discomfort. So I tried to surround that physical feeling with my focus.

FACILITATOR: What did you notice about that?

PARTICIPANT 2: I sort of forgot about it.

FACILITATOR: So maybe the first reaction is to scratch . . .

PARTICIPANT 2: Yeah, almost automatically!

FACILITATOR: Is that how you typically respond to itches? Observe them for a bit? Or was this different?

PARTICIPANT 2: At first, I almost reached to scratch it, like I normally would. Then I just stayed with the feeling instead. Then I went back to the breath, then sort of forgot about it. I don't know, my focus just changed.

PARTICIPANT 3: The more I practice, the more I find that my thoughts do still wander but they tend to come back much more quickly. Early on I had trouble keeping my thoughts from running away, and now it's easier to come back to the moment again.

FACILITATOR: So for you, too, you're noticing that the mind still does its thing, it still wanders off. But you're increasingly able to notice that and to catch it sooner, and to intentionally bring focus back to the present experience.

So we're hearing about some changes that people are noticing. Anyone noticing that their experience is pretty similar to what it was like in Session 1? That things aren't really changing?

PARTICIPANT 3: Well, I find that focusing on breathing just helps me come back. It doesn't really help me keep from wandering, but focusing on the breath helps me come back. It's the one constant; it's like a home base. That part is easier.

FACILITATOR: As many of you are describing, and as we have been talking about since the first week, the point is not to keep our minds from wandering. They will wander; it's what minds do. The idea is to notice, and to practice bringing the attention back, again and again. To realize maybe we have some choice in how we respond to what our minds are doing. And that might get easier with practice. We'll see.

Often by this fourth week, people begin noticing some changes in how they are responding to these physical, emotional, or cognitive experiences that arise not only in their practice but in daily life situations.

PARTICIPANT 1: This practice is helping me deal with my wife's drinking. I usually get really upset.

FACILITATOR: What are you noticing that's different?

PARTICIPANT 1: It's helping me focus in on what my emotions are.

FACILITATOR: So in that moment when you typically get upset, what are you noticing?

PARTICIPANT 1: I'm not as quick to act on my anger or judge.

FACILITATOR: So you notice that anger coming up, and then how are you responding to it?

PARTICIPANT 1: What I do now that is kind of surprising is that, instead of yelling, I make sure she is okay and safe, and I feel more compassion.

FACILITATOR: That's interesting, thank you. What are others' experiences?

PARTICIPANT 2: I'm noticing some similar things. It's not anger for me, it's the ability to take a moment and focus on what the real issue might be, what I'm really feeling, how it's affecting me emotionally and in my body. Maybe I am more aware when I start to get caught up in something, then when I start to notice it, I am aware of my mind taking off. Then I just sort of stop and refocus.

FACILITATOR: Yes, and that's the practice right there, to be aware, just noticing that your mind is wandering or "taking off," and maybe stopping right there and intentionally bringing the focus back to the present. Great.

INDIVIDUAL AND COMMON RELAPSE RISKS

One of the primary intentions of this session is to shift from integration of mindfulness into daily life to a specific focus on how these practices might be useful in challenging or high-risk situations. Each of us has situations in which we tend to behave reactively, whether reaching for a substance, lashing out at someone, or withdrawing. This exercise in identifying challenging situations not only helps with the recognition of areas that are risky for each individual but highlights reactive patterns common to many of us.

We typically begin by asking participants to share some recent or typical triggers or risky situations. They might refer to the Noticing Triggers Worksheet from

Session 2 (Handout 2.2) to identify common triggers, or reflect on past lapses or challenging situations. We ask for the general experience or type of situation rather than the story (e.g., categories such as conflict with family, situations or settings in which they would use substances, or feelings of anger or loneliness). Writing participants' responses on the whiteboard can be helpful in this exercise. As several examples of challenging situations or triggers are identified, common groupings or categories often emerge. It can be useful to refer at this point to the research on common precipitants of relapse. In the groups we have worked with thus far, the "top three" categories have reliably emerged: negative emotional states ("negative" is traditionally used in the relapse prevention/CBT practice; we often refer to them as "challenging"); social pressure (including social situations associated with substance use that do not necessarily involve direct peer pressure but in which there are felt pressures to use); and interpersonal conflict (often with a family member or partner). Highlighting these categories can bring awareness both to an individual's unique risk patterns and to the commonality of these challenges among all of us.

SOBER SPACE IN A CHALLENGING SITUATION

The in-session practice of the SOBER space in a challenging situation (Practice 4.3) allows participants to move from discussion of these situations to working with the experiences more directly. Similar to urge surfing, the SOBER space is a way to practice pausing right at the brink of where we usually become reactive, breaking the inertia of automatic pilot and bringing awareness to whatever is arising. The intention isn't to change or "fix" how we are feeling or thinking, but to observe the experience just as it is and allow the space necessary to make a more mindful, intentional choice in the midst of discomfort or reactivity. This rationale is repeatedly offered to participants and in our experience is never overemphasized.

We ask participants to pick a recent situation in which they were triggered or behaved reactively, or to imagine one from the list on the whiteboard. In selecting a scenario with which to practice, we request that people choose something that is not going to be too overwhelming or difficult, but that provides a sufficient challenge in their lives (a 3 or 4 on a scale of 10). Participants often have trouble picking the "right" or "best" scenario. Any situation that elicits a reaction will provide material with which to practice. The situation or feeling that comes to mind first is often a good choice.

In addition to inquiring about the experience after the exercise, it can be helpful to discuss integrating this practice into daily life. For example, what would it be like to do this in a difficult situation? What would make it hard to do this practice in these situations? How might you work with that, or how might you remember to do this practice? In what situations can you imagine this being a useful practice for you?

WALKING MEDITATION

There are several ways to practice walking meditation (Practice 4.4). As with all of the practices, this meditation is best led from experience. Facilitators might narrate the process they are engaging in while doing the walking meditation themselves. Again, we provide an example at the end of the chapter, but it is our hope that facilitators will not use this as a script, but will lead from their own experience.

Walking meditation can be led as a formal, structured, traditional practice (using silent labels such as "lifting, placing, shifting") or as a more open awareness of the whole process, allowing a curious, even childlike quality (What is it like to walk? What do the feet feel like as they move? Notice all the muscles it takes to move the leg). The facilitator might offer playful suggestions, such as imagining walking for the first time, as though we have just dropped into this human body and our job is only to observe it as it walks.

Participants can experiment with different speeds. To begin, one might walk at a pace that is slower than usual to give oneself a better chance to become fully aware of the sensations of walking. Once participants feel comfortable walking slowly with awareness, they might experiment with walking at faster speeds. If agitation or restlessness arise, it might be helpful to begin walking faster, with awareness, and to slow down naturally as the mind settles.

Walking meditation can be done "formally," in one's home or an appropriate outdoor area, or "informally" outside or in public, in day-to-day life. The practice can be a way to check in while walking to work or to the bus stop—simply note how the body feels, returning repeatedly to physical sensations of walking.

Often people feel awkward, silly, or self-conscious while doing this practice. Awareness of these reactions, too, is part of the practice. It can be helpful to include all of this when leading the exercise, encouraging participants to notice whatever arises, including any thoughts they are having about the exercise, or feelings of embarrassment or silliness, and then returning focus again on the experience of walking.

When possible, we lead the group through the initial instructions and then have them move into a larger area to practice on their own for a while. We encourage participants to pick a short length of ground and walk the length of that course, turn, and walk back in the opposite direction. The idea is to experience just walking versus trying to get somewhere. In certain settings, it is not possible to walk back and forth or to leave the room to practice, in which case we might stay in the room and walk in a circle or in whatever format works.

For people for whom walking is inaccessible or not possible, they can participate in any way is appropriate. Keeping the intention of the practice in mind, facilitators can suggest other mindful movements, or any practices that bring attention to the experience of the body engaging in typical daily movements.

DAILY PRACTICE

Following this fourth week, we ask clients to again practice the sitting meditation or body scan, whichever they choose (Handout 4.1). They are asked to practice the walking meditation at least twice and the SOBER space in routine daily experiences and/or when they experience a challenging situation or emotion. Participants are also asked to record their meditation practice using the Daily Practice Tracking Sheet (Handout 4.2).

CLOSING

The session may close with a few moments of silence or with a one- to two-word description of present-moment experience, as done at the beginning of the session.

Awareness of Seeing
PRACTICE 4.1

Intentions

+ Observing present experience through a different "sense door"

+ Noticing deeply habitual ways in which the mind works (i.e., "automatically" labeling and categorizing) and how this can obstruct our true vision or raw experience

+ What's actually happening versus what the mind thinks it already "knows"

Sit or stand so that you can comfortably see out the window (if available). Take a few moments to look outside (or around the room), noticing all the different sights. The colors, the different textures, the shapes. For the next few minutes, see if you can let go of trying to make sense of things in the way that we usually do and instead can see them as merely patterns of color, shapes, and movement.

There is no need to analyze or think about what you are seeing . . . as best you can, just experience seeing. If your mind wanders, or you are having thoughts such as "This is weird" or "I can't do this," see if you can notice that as well, with gentleness, and bring your attention back to the experience of seeing.

Whenever you become aware that you have started to think about what is being seen, or the mind begins telling stories about what you are seeing rather than simply experiencing it, gently let go of your involvement with these thoughts and arrive again at this experience of simply seeing what is here: the colors, the shapes, lines and edges, movement.

When you are ready, bringing your focus back into the room if you are looking outside or expand your focus to include the room you are in and the people around you if you have been focusing on sights inside the room.

Sitting Meditation
Sound, Breath, Sensation, Thought
PRACTICE 4.2

Intentions

+ Expanding the field of awareness to include other sensory experiences

+ Being aware that all experiences are in the same class, rather than thoughts or emotions being more "important" or personal than sound, and that all these experiences arise and pass in our field of awareness

+ Practicing observation of physical and emotional discomfort and meeting it with patience, curiosity, and kindness, rather than with resistance

+ Further noticing the mind's tendency to automatically label, categorize, and judge

---

Settle into a comfortable sitting position. If you are in a chair, maybe placing your feet flat on the floor with your legs uncrossed. Gently allow your eyes to close, or if you choose to leave them open, rest your gaze on a spot a few feet in front of you. Finding your posture, sitting with a sense of dignity, so you are alert and awake and also relaxed.

Feeling the weight of your body in the chair or on your cushion. Noticing the places where your body makes contact with the floor and with your chair.

Maybe taking a moment to remember your intention for being here and committing to being present as best you can for the duration of this practice. Finding that gentle determination to stay with this practice, knowing that you can let go and begin again as often as you need to.

Now just releasing whatever your mind might have come into this group with today. Letting go of the past, of planning or worrying about the future. For now, your job is simply to relax into the present, releasing thoughts as many times as you need to, and beginning again with attention to the present experience.

Let's begin by simply noticing sound and the sensation of hearing. Observing the sounds inside your body and the sounds outside your body. Noticing the texture and the pitch of the sounds. Maybe listening for the quietest or most distant sound. If you find yourself carried away at any time from the experience of hearing, just noting that and gently guiding your attention back to sound. Rather than reaching to hear sounds, allowing them to come to you.

Now allowing the different sounds to fade into the background of your awareness, and resting attention on breathing, the sensations in your abdomen as the breath moves in and out of your body. There is no need to try to control or change the breathing in any way—simply observe your body breathing. Maybe you notice the feeling of air coming in and out of the nostrils, or the slight stretching as your abdomen rises with each inbreath and gently falls with each outbreath. Focusing your attention gently and firmly on the sensations of each inbreath and each outbreath.

When your attention wanders off the breath, just noticing that and gently guiding it back. Letting go and beginning again, with your attention resting on the breath.

Now when you're ready, allowing the sensations of breath to fade into the background of your experience and bringing your attention to other sensations in the body. Noticing all the different sensations that may be present in this moment—sensations of touch,

(continued)

105

pressure, tingling, pulsing, itching, or whatever it may be. Spend a few moments exploring these sensations. You might scan the body, from the toes up to the head, or just open your awareness to the body as a whole, noticing whatever arises and letting your attention go to that sensation or area.

If you find sensations that are particularly intense, maybe bringing your awareness to these areas and exploring with gentleness and curiosity the detailed pattern of sensations there: What do the sensations feel like? Do they vary over time? Continuing to observe the sensations in your body for a few more moments.

When you notice that your awareness is no longer on the body, noting what is on your mind and then gently congratulating yourself; you have already come back and are once more aware of your experience. And beginning again.

Now when you are ready, allowing the sensations in your body to move into the background of your awareness, and shifting your attention to thoughts. See if you can notice the next thought that arises in the mind. Now as best you can, watching each thought as it arises and passes away, noticing them as they arise, then gently letting them pass.

You might try labeling this process of thinking, simply saying to yourself "thought" or "thinking" as each thought comes. If you notice yourself pulled into a thought or story, just observing that as well and gently letting go, returning your attention again to the awareness of thinking, to watching your mind. If you notice your attention repeatedly getting pulled into thoughts, you can always reconnect with the here and now by bringing your awareness back to the movements of breathing. Continuing to practice this on your own for a few more moments.

As we close this meditation, reflecting back on how this practice was for you. Noticing if there is any judgment about how you did. And trusting that anytime we bring mindful attention to our experience, anytime we stop and have the intention of coming into the present, we are taking care of ourselves in a very fundamental way, no matter what comes up during the practice or what our minds and bodies are doing.

Now gently, as you are ready, gently allowing your eyes to open and allowing your awareness to include the room.

SOBER Space in a Challenging Situation
PRACTICE 4.3

Intentions

+ Pausing at the brink of where we typically become reactive and practicing presence and awareness

+ Learning that it is possible to "stay" with an experience, even when it feels intolerable

+ Exploring our experience with curiosity and kindness

+ Experiencing how greater awareness can allow space necessary to make a more mindful, intentional choice

---

Next we are going to do an exercise similar to the SOBER space practice we did last week, taking it one step further. Again, the SOBER space is a practice that you can do almost anywhere, anytime, because it is brief and simple. It can be used in the midst of a high-risk or stressful situation, if you are upset about something, when you are experiencing urges and cravings to use, or just throughout the day as a way to return to your present experience.

Can anyone review what the steps are?

Stop, or **shift** out of automatic pilot and into awareness, in whatever situation you find yourself in. This is the first step in freeing yourself from the automatic pilot mode. Stopping or shifting focus to direct inner experience in itself can be a powerful step in making changes in your life.

Observe what is happening right now, in this very moment—sensations, thoughts, emotions.

Bring your attention to sensations of **breathing**.

Expand your awareness again to include a sense of your whole experience—sensation, thoughts and emotions.

Respond mindfully, with awareness of the many choices in front of you in this situation. What is it you really need? How can you best take care of yourself in this moment?

For this exercise, we're going to ask you to picture yourself in a situation in which you might be tempted to react in a way that is not in your best interest. But we are going to ask you to imagine, as you did a few weeks ago when we practiced urge surfing, that you do not use or react in this way. You might imagine a scenario in which you react in a way that feels automatic or reactive, for instance, a relationship or a situation where you might react with anger or in a way that's hurtful to you or another person, or one that elicits craving or urges for substances. It's best to pick something challenging but not overwhelming. Choose something you are comfortable working with. We encourage you to stay with whatever comes up with a sense of gentleness and curiosity. If this feels like something you do not want to do or are not ready to do, respect that limit.

Does anyone need a little more time to think of something?

Okay, let's practice this now:

Closing your eyes, if that feels comfortable for you, or finding a soft focus a few feet in front of you on the floor. Now bringing to mind this situation or circumstance that has been, or you imagine might be, challenging for you. Take a moment to imagine that person,

(continued)

place, situation, or feeling now. Really putting yourself in that story, playing it out right up until the point where you feel that discomfort or reactivity.

So the first step is to **stop,** right there at that challenging point, and make the choice to step out of automatic pilot by shifting your awareness to your internal experience.

The next step is to **observe,** becoming really aware of what is happening with you right now, first noticing physical sensations, what is happening in the body. Then noticing any thoughts that might be arising. Then noticing what emotions are present. Noticing, too, any urges you might have to act in a certain way. We're not pushing anything away or forcing anything out, just acknowledge what is happening for you.

The third step is to gather our attention in and let it just rest on sensations of **breathing,** aware of the movements of the abdomen, the rise and fall of each breath. Just using the anchor of the breath to come into the body and stay present.

Now, having gathered our attention, the next step is to **expand** this awareness to include a sense of the entire body, heart, and mind, including any tightness or tension, emotion, checking in again with the mind and any thoughts or urges. Holding your entire body in this slightly softer, more spacious awareness.

From this place of greater awareness, notice once again the situation that you are in . . . the situation, the emotion, or the person that is risky for you. And look at the choices you have in front of you. Notice that no matter what thoughts and sensations are going through your mind or body right now, you still have the choices of how to **respond.** From this place of awareness and compassion for yourself, ask yourself what the best choice is for you, what is most in line with how you want to be in this life, with what is truly important to you. Imagine yourself making that choice, one that leads you away from reacting in any way that is harmful to you or others. As you make this choice, notice again what is happening in your body. What sensations, thoughts, and feelings are here?

When you are ready, gently letting that scene go, allowing your attention to return to this room, allowing your eyes to open.

Walking Meditation
PRACTICE 4.4

Intentions

+ Bringing attention to the body in motion, grounding in physical sensations
+ Increasing awareness of another often "automatic" daily activity
+ Noticing the experience of just walking versus trying to get somewhere

For this practice, we will have our eyes open. Begin by standing with your knees soft and arms just resting comfortably at your sides. Letting your focus be soft, maybe just resting on the ground a few feet in front of you. Now bringing awareness to the bottoms of your feet, sensing the physical sensations of where they contact the floor, and sensing the weight of your body being supported by your legs and feet.

Now allowing your weight to shift very gently over to the left side, so that the left leg is bearing the weight and the right leg is light. Feeling how the left leg becomes "full" and the right leg sort of empties out. Now shifting the weight back to center, noticing how the body knows where that is. Maybe noticing if there are any urges to shift to the other side. Now allowing the weight to shift to the right, transferring the weight onto the right leg.

Now very slowly taking a step with the left leg, staying with all the sensations as you do this. Feeling the left heel come off the floor, the muscles contracting, the joints moving. Placing that foot down on the floor in front of you and allowing the weight to shift a little onto that foot. Pausing here for a moment. Noticing if there are any urges present—maybe to move the right leg.

And then moving the right leg—lifting the heel and moving the leg forward, placing the heel and then the whole foot on the ground, then shifting the weight forward onto the right leg.

Continuing in this way, lifting the leg, moving it forward, placing it on the ground. Being aware, as best you can, of physical sensations in the feet and legs and of the contact of the feet with the floor. Keeping your gaze directed softly ahead. You might label the movements of each step as a way to focus your attention: "lifting, moving, placing." Or you might allow your attention to move throughout the body as we do in the body scan, noticing all the sensations as you move.

As with the other meditations we have practiced, your attention will likely wander at some point to thoughts about this practice or to plans, memories, whatever. When you notice this, just gently let those release and allow the attention to fall back onto the present experience of walking.

Now when you are ready, make your way back to your chair, keeping the same quality of awareness as you take your seat.

Mindfulness in Challenging Situations
HANDOUT 4.1

THEME

Mindfulness practice can help foster a sense of spaciousness and perspective in challenging situations. In this session, we focus on staying present in situations that have previously triggered substance use or other reactive behaviors. We learn how we might relate differently to pressures or urges to react or use, and practice responding with awareness rather than reacting "automatically" or out of habit.

INTEGRATING PRACTICE INTO YOUR WEEK

1. Practice sitting meditation or body scan each day, as best you can.

2. Practice the SOBER space regularly and whenever you notice challenging emotions, sensations, and urges, or anytime you notice yourself becoming reactive. Note your practice on the Daily Practice Tracking Sheet.

3. Practice the walking meditation at least once this week. The purpose of the walking practice is to connect with awareness of the body while in motion and in day-to-day life. You can practice this formally in a private space, walking back and forth along a short path. You might also practice this informally in your daily routine, for example, when walking to the bus stop or walking your dog. If practicing in daily life, you may experiment with moving your attention between sensations of walking, the experience of seeing, the experience of hearing, and observation of the breath, resting your awareness on each for a few moments and continuing to move between them.

Instructions: Each day, record your mindfulness practice, also noting any barriers, observations, or comments.

Day/ date	Formal practice: How long? Which practices?	SOBER space	Walking	Notes/comments
	____ minutes	How often? In what situations?	How many times?	
	____ minutes	How often? In what situations?	How many times?	
	____ minutes	How often? In what situations?	How many times?	
	____ minutes	How often? In what situations?	How many times?	
	____ minutes	How often? In what situations?	How many times?	
	____ minutes	How often? In what situations?	How many times?	
	____ minutes	How often? In what situations?	How many times?	

SESSION 5

Acceptance and Skillful Action

Grant me the serenity
To accept the things I cannot change;
The courage to change the things I can;
And the wisdom to know the difference.
—REINHOLD NIEBUHR

Materials

- Bell
- Whiteboard/markers
- Handout 5.1: Using the SOBER Space in Challenging Situations Worksheet
- Handout 5.2: Session 5 Theme and Daily Practice: Acceptance and Skillful Action
- Handout 5.3: Daily Practice Tracking Sheet
- Audio Files: Sitting Meditation (Sound, Breath, Sensation, Thought, Emotion), Mindful Movement

Theme

In this session, we are exploring acceptance of what arises while also encouraging healthy action in participants' lives. We might not have control over things that happen to us, emotions that arise, current job or family situations, or other people's behaviors and reactions. When we fight against these things, however, we tend to feel frustrated, angry, or defeated, which can be triggers for substance use or other reactive behaviors. When we accept the present as it is, we are not being passive. We are allowing what *already is true* without struggle or resistance. This is often a necessary first step toward change. The same is true of self-acceptance; it often requires a complete acceptance of ourselves just as we are before real change can occur.

Goals

- Introduce and cultivate a different relationship toward challenging experiences, such as uncomfortable sensations, emotions, or situations.

- Discuss the role of acceptance in the change process.

- Introduce mindful movement as another way to practice awareness and acceptance.

Session Outline

- Check-In
- Sitting Meditation: Sound, Breath, Sensation, Thought, Emotion (Practice 5.1)
- Practice Review
- Discussion of Acceptance and Skillful Action
- SOBER Space (in Pairs) (Practice 5.2)
- Using the SOBER Space in Challenging Situations Worksheet
- Mindful Movement
- Daily Practice
- Closing

Practice for This Week

- Daily Practice Tracking Sheet
- Sitting Meditation, Mindful Movement, or Body Scan
- SOBER Space, regularly and when you find yourself in a challenging or high-risk situation
- Using the SOBER Space in Challenging Situations Worksheet

CHECK-IN

Participants may be invited to share one or two words describing their present-moment physical sensations, mind states, or feelings/emotions.

SITTING MEDITATION: SOUND, BREATH, SENSATION, THOUGHT, EMOTION

The meditation in Session 5 (Practice 5.1) focuses on awareness of sound, breath, body sensations, thought, and emotion. There is a specific focus on discomfort or any experience that is associated with resistance or tension. This opening meditation lays the foundation for the session's focus on acceptance of all experience, whether pleasant or unpleasant, invited or uninvited.

The use of poetry in meditation instruction and practice has a long and rich tradition. Often poetry can open doors and deepen understandings, complementing the meditation instruction offered by teachers or facilitators. We sometimes use poetry at the end of the meditation in Session 4, and throughout the course, if and when it feels helpful in conveying the essence of a particular practice. Here we include Rumi's poem "The Guest House," which is often used in MBSR and MBCT, to convey the intention of inviting all present experience in as a teacher or guide. Rumi suggests going beyond merely accepting or tolerating challenging experiences to "greeting them at the door, laughing." Discussion following this meditation might include responses to this poem, and specifically to the idea of appreciatively welcoming all experience, whether it is pleasant, unpleasant, or neutral, because it may provide an opportunity for further discovery and growth.

PRACTICE REVIEW

Participants may notice at this point in the course that they are repeatedly meeting the same challenges, and perhaps experiencing doubt regarding whether or not they are "able" to meditate. It can be very useful to review the five common meditation challenges (restlessness, sleepiness or dullness, craving, aversion, and doubt). We remind participants that these are challenges that have been experienced for thousands of years and are thus very impersonal; these experiences just tend to arise when we ask the mind to maintain awareness, focus, and presence. Facilitators might suggest naming these challenges when they arise in meditation: for example, "Okay, doubt is here" or "This is sleepiness. What does sleepiness feel like?"

Discussion of the SOBER space often centers on whether or not participants have remembered to implement this practice in stressful and/or nonstressful situations, and what they noticed. Again, we often hear comments about this practice "working" or "not working," reflecting the enduring misperception that meditation is supposed to "fix" something. It is helpful to remain aware of this theme and gently bring attention to it when it arises in discussion.

Participants were also asked to practice walking meditation over the previous week. Again, the focus in this practice, and thus the discussion, is similar to that of the other practices: bringing attention to the experience, whatever it is, and addressing any barriers to practice. People often have experiences with walking meditation that differ from their experiences with sitting meditation. This is neither good nor bad, and allows an opportunity to note differences in how the mind responds to the various modes of practice. Issues that sometimes arise with walking meditation are diffusion of focus, feeling "spacey," and feeling embarrassed or silly. Others, however, find it easier to focus while moving than while sitting relatively still in the sitting practices. Participants are encouraged to notice these experiences, too, as part of the practice. It may be helpful for maintaining focus in walking meditation to return attention to sensations on the bottom of the feet when focus becomes diffuse. Clients might also practice switching from seeing to hearing, to sensation, and to thought, or to hold attention on "lifting, moving, and placing" of the feet as a way to focus attention. Participants might play with these different techniques and see what works best for them.

SOBER SPACE (IN PAIRS)

The SOBER space (Practice 5.2) is practiced in a somewhat different way in this session. The group breaks off into dyads, and partners are asked to engage in a brief informal conversation with each other about a typical daily hassle, stressor, or something that tends to trigger a reaction. We often suggest a topic that most people can relate to, such as transportation issues (e.g., being cut off in traffic, parking hassles, unreliable bus schedules). When it seems as though participants have become sufficiently involved in their conversation, the facilitator rings the bell. Upon hearing the bell, participants are asked to stop wherever they are, even if in midsentence. The facilitator then guides them through a brief SOBER space.

Introducing this interpersonal element—the potential anxiety of having to interact with peers—and the stress associated with daily hassles can help generalize the SOBER practice to a broader class of experiences and contexts. Tension, anxiety, and automatic reactions and behaviors may arise in this exercise, providing the opportunity to observe how rapidly these states can emerge even when simply talking *about* a stressor, and to practice the SOBER space in a slightly more agitated, distracted, or automatic mode.

Discussion of this exercise often centers on noticing experience, with attention to differences before and after the SOBER space. Facilitators may ask about ways in which participants would engage with their partner if they were to return to the conversation following this practice, and to notice whether this is different from how they previously engaged. It can be useful to inquire, too, about how what they experienced in the exercise is similar to or different from ways in which they typically interact in their daily lives.

FACILITATOR: What did people notice?

PARTICIPANT: I noticed that as I was telling my story I was getting back into that same moment again, like I was right back there, and getting upset, and thinking that I shouldn't be upset.

FACILITATOR: So you noticed yourself feeling upset even just telling the story, then the thought "I shouldn't be upset"?

PARTICIPANT: Yeah, that was a thought I had when I heard the bell.

FACILITATOR: What else did you notice?

PARTICIPANT: I was getting heated.

FACILITATOR: Heated—what did you experience?

PARTICIPANT: I was getting angry, getting tense, and I wasn't really breathing.

FACILITATOR: Okay, so when I rang the bell, you noticed anger, some tension and shallow breathing, and the thought "I shouldn't be getting upset."

PARTICIPANT: Yeah. I was like this. (*Tenses body.*) I didn't really notice it while I was talking to my partner here, just when you rang the bell. I sort of dropped in and was like, wow, I am really tense and angry. Then I thought, "Wait, it's over, it's okay."

FACILITATOR: Hmm. Is this familiar at all to you? Do you experience this tension and emotion when relaying a story to someone or maybe just reviewing an event in your mind?

PARTICIPANT: (*Laughs.*) Oh, yeah. I get all worked up over something in my head, and I don't even realize it.

FACILITATOR: Okay, thank you. So we can see in this exercise how easy it can be to forget these mindfulness skills and get pretty worked up over something that's not even happening. This exercise might be a little closer to how we're usually engaged in day-to-day life and how quickly we lose awareness of our experience. It can be especially challenging to stay present and aware in interpersonal situations, as you might have just experienced. What is it like, right in the middle of an interaction or experience, to just stop and notice?

USING THE SOBER SPACE IN CHALLENGING SITUATIONS

The Using the SOBER Space in Challenging Situations Worksheet (Handout 5.1) can be introduced following the SOBER space as an extension of this exercise into everyday life. Participants are asked to identify high-risk situations they encounter throughout the week, again recognizing the different components of their reactions. The emphasis is on identifying specific experiences, whether physical, emotional, or cognitive, that might serve as cues for practicing the SOBER space. For example, a participant might notice that his breathing changes and his ears begin to feel hot as his anger escalates. These physiological experiences, once identified, might be a useful cue for him to stop and observe his experience. He might bring his focus to his breath for a few moments to gather and ground his attention, and then expand awareness again to his broader experience, and perhaps to the situation he is in. Finally, he might respond a little more intentionally, with greater awareness of his choices in that moment rather than in the habitual manner in which he might typically react.

It is useful to walk through an example in session using the worksheet, identifying specific cues and including ideas of how using the SOBER space might affect the experience and response in a particular situation.

DISCUSSION OF ACCEPTANCE AND SKILLFUL ACTION

A fundamental part of the practices included in the course is learning to *recognize and accept the present moment as it is,* and bring attention to our reactions to what has arisen. As we begin to release our struggle with the parts of reality over which we don't have control, we stop resisting what is true. This letting go can free us from an unwinnable struggle, allowing greater flexibility and space to see more clearly and to make real and effective changes. It allows us the freedom to respond instead of react.

As practice becomes deeper and further integrated into our lives, we may begin noticing when we are meeting experience with aversion, attempting to suppress or control what is happening versus acknowledging and allowing an experience, whether or not it is what we wanted. Perhaps we even begin to welcome these challenging experiences with friendliness and curiosity.

The inquiry around acceptance and its relationship to change often emerges organically at this point in the course and is a natural extension of the "Guest House" poem at the end of the sitting practice. In our experience, the form this discussion has taken has been somewhat different with each group but has centered on the same basic theme. Again, facilitators elicit ideas and themes from the group rather than "teaching" a concept. The following is one example:

FACILITATOR: Up to this point, we have talked a lot about being aware of and accepting physical sensations, thoughts, and emotions, including those that are uncomfortable. We've focused on noticing our experience, and not necessarily *doing* anything, just noticing, raising our awareness of our experience as it is. So where does change fit in? If we just accept everything, how does anything ever change?

PARTICIPANT: Well, you need awareness of what's coming at you, knowing that you can't change a lot of it and so you might as well accept it instead of being miserable and obsessing about it. Because then you just get angry. Like there was this guy who cut in line in front of me at the coffee shop yesterday. I could have gotten really angry and thought about how to get back at him, maybe in the parking lot. I'd get all worked up without even noticing, and what good does that do?

FACILITATOR: So what are you accepting here?

PARTICIPANT: His attitude and that people don't act the way I want them to. That I can't change him, so trying to get back at him is pointless.

FACILITATOR: How about what's coming up for you in that situation? Does acceptance come in there?

PARTICIPANT: Oh, yeah. I guess I can choose to accept that I am angry, because I just am. But then I can choose how to deal with that, how I want to respond instead of just flying off the handle.

FACILITATOR: This reminds me of the serenity prayer. Who here is familiar with it?

> Grant me the serenity
> To accept the things I cannot change;
> The courage to change the things I can;
> And the wisdom to know the difference.

So what are we accepting?

PARTICIPANT: What we can't control.

FACILITATOR: Like what?

PARTICIPANT: Oh—like other people, or the past, or even what I am feeling.

FACILITATOR: So the acceptance of what is *already here*. What's arrived here in front of us in this moment has already arrived; it's here. We can't change that. As you said, that might be a situation, like someone cutting you off in line, or an emotion that comes up, like anger. And we can spend a lot of energy fighting what's already here: "It shouldn't be like this. I hate this. Why is it like this?" or "I shouldn't feel anger." Where does that get us?

PARTICIPANT: It makes us frustrated, angry, stuck. Sick.

For many of us, acceptance suggests a passive stance. The intention in this session is to help participants recognize that by meeting an experience with openness and honesty, seeing it as it really is, we are giving ourselves a genuine choice in how we respond. We shift from reacting without awareness, or with aversion, to responding with a greater sense of space, choice, and compassion. The following is a continuation of the prior dialogue:

> FACILITATOR: So this automatic, reactive behavior we've been talking about and working with over the past several weeks often comes from resisting, or nonacceptance, of what is actually happening in this moment. We reject what already *is* because it isn't what we think it *should* be. We are fighting against something we can't change.
>
> PARTICIPANT: First, we have to acknowledge and accept, I guess, what's in front of us. Then we can make a choice about how we want to respond.
>
> FACILITATOR: Yes. It allows us to start from where we actually are (versus where we wish we were or where we think we should be) and go from there. A common misconception is that acceptance is passive, that we're letting people or circumstances walk all over us. What do you think about that?
>
> PARTICIPANT: No. It seems like accepting things as they are would allow us to make better choices.
>
> FACILITATOR: Yes. We're not talking about accepting being victimized; it's a kinder attitude toward ourselves and our experience so that we can choose how we act in the world as opposed to just "reacting." This doesn't mean we have to like it. We are learning to stay with it and make a more intentional choice about where to go from here instead of just reacting. So maybe accepting how things are gives us the ability to change.

Working with anger, whether deep-seated hatred or rage, or more subtle forms such as impatience or irritation, often arises as part of the discussion of acceptance and skillful action. Anger can be a powerful emotional state with a decentering quality that can elicit reactive behavior. As explored in the previous dialogue, bringing awareness and curiosity to the experience of anger, rather than immediately reacting to it or attempting to suppress it, can help acknowledge its presence and shift attention to the *experience* of the anger rather than to the object of the anger. Bringing attention to the body and physical experience not only may diffuse its charge, but often reveals other emotions such as hurt, vulnerability, anxiety, and fear that can underlie the anger. It can be a powerful way to show us the places where we're stuck or hurting. We often include this as part of this session's discussion, using concrete examples of situations that have evoked anger for participants.

MINDFUL MOVEMENT

Mindful movement provides another opportunity to practice mindful attention. Just as in sitting meditation when we observe sensations of the breath, in mindful movement, we bring attention to the sensations in the body while moving, stretching, and engaging in different postures. Some facilitators may be intimidated by mindful movement if they confuse it with yoga or assume it requires certain physical abilities. While there may be overlap between mindful movement and some yoga practices, the intention of mindful movement is very simple. Just as with walking meditation, the purpose is to bring awareness to the body while it is moving. In doing this, there is an opportunity to notice the subtle interactions of body and mind. The movements are slow and gentle, allowing time to notice everything from the intention to move to the sensations created by the movement and the reactions of the mind. Participants may notice the urge to speed up and rush ahead. Facilitators might also ask if they notice comparing and judging and remind them to gently redirect attention to physical sensation in the body as it moves.

As such, the specific movements or postures are not important, so we don't prescribe them here. What is important is that the practice is accessible to everyone in the room. Facilitators begin by encouraging participants to respect what's most appropriate for their own body today, and to modify any of the suggested movements appropriately.

Although the presentation and practice of mindful movement varies with the experience and preferences of the facilitators, it is always critical to begin by emphasizing self-care and checking in regarding any physical limitations. Facilitators may choose a few postures that are comfortable for them and suitable for the group. We often encourage facilitators to use positions and movements that they themselves enjoy. The postures are less important than the quality of attention brought to the practice. Typically, we try a few very simple postures in session that may be done sitting or standing, or on the floor if appropriate for the group and setting.

As with other practices, this, too, is followed by an inquiry into participants' experiences. Facilitators might suggest this practice as another way to become aware of sensations in the body and to practice noticing the wandering mind. Emotional responses may arise as well, because many participants have difficult histories and relationships with their bodies. The practice can also facilitate greater awareness of and a gentle approach to these difficulties, learning to befriend the body, allowing space for emotional and physical discomfort. There may be awareness, too, of the pleasant sensations and the sense of well-being that often arise in mindful movement.

DAILY PRACTICE

Following this fifth week, clients are given the choice to practice the sitting meditation, body scan, or mindful movement. We suggest that they continue practicing the SOBER space and complete the Using the SOBER Space in Challenging Situations Worksheet (Handout 5.1). This worksheet helps identify potential cues for taking a SOBER space in situations that might elicit habitual, reactive behaviors. Participants are also asked to record their meditation practice on the Daily Practice Tracking Sheet (Handout 5.3).

CLOSING

As practiced in previous sessions, the session ends with a few moments of silence and sharing a one- to two-word description of present-moment experience.

Sitting Meditation
Sound, Breath, Sensation, Thought, Emotion
PRACTICE 5.1

Intentions

✦ Relating to emotion as another arising (and passing) event, with sensory and cognitive elements

✦ Noticing raw elements of emotions versus stories about it or reactivity to it

---

Take a few minutes now to settle into your chair, finding a posture that feels relaxed, centered, and dignified. Allow your eyes to close if that's comfortable for you. Feeling the weight of your body—where it contacts the chair or your cushion, where your feet or legs contact the ground. The points of contact your body makes with itself—maybe your hands resting on your legs or your arms against your sides. Maybe you can feel the places where your clothing touches your skin.

Now bringing your attention to sounds, and to the sensation of hearing. You might observe sounds both inside and outside the body, both near and far away.

Noticing the texture and the pitch of the sounds. Noticing how the often mind labels or makes sense of these sounds. Staying as best you can with the raw experience of hearing rather than the thoughts and ideas. As thoughts arise, returning again and again to the experience of hearing. And if you find yourself carried away from awareness of hearing, just noting that and gently guiding your attention back to the experience of receiving these sounds.

Now letting the different sounds fade into the background of your awareness and allowing your attention to shift to your breath. The inbreath, perhaps a slight pause, the outbreath. Aware of the sensations in your abdomen as the breath moves in and out of your body. Noticing that your body knows exactly what to do. Just observing as your body breathes, the air as it flows in and out of the nostrils, or slight stretching as your abdomen rises, or the expansion of the chest with the inbreath, and the gentle falling with the outbreath. As best you can, staying with the sensations of each breath as it enters and leaves the body. Each time you notice that your mind has wandered off the breath, gently letting go and beginning again, allowing your attention to return to sensations of breathing.

Now when you're ready, allowing the breath to fade into the background of your awareness and shifting your attention to other the sensations in the body. Noticing all the different sensations that may be present: sensations of touch, pressure, tingling, pulsing, itching, or whatever it may be. Spending a few moments exploring these sensations.

If there are sensations that are particularly intense or uncomfortable, bringing your awareness to these areas and seeing if you can stay with them, breathing into these areas and exploring with gentleness and curiosity the detailed pattern of sensations: What do these sensations really feel like? Do they stay the same, or do they change? Is there a way to experience this discomfort without resisting or fighting it? Noticing any reactions that arise, and meeting whatever is here with kindness. If there is tension, softening around those areas as best you can. Seeing now if you can just allow whatever is here to just be.

Now allowing the focus of your attention to shift from sensations to awareness of thoughts. Seeing if you can notice the very next thought that arises in the mind. Then

(continued)

122

just watching each thought as it appears and passes away. If you notice yourself getting involved or lost in a thought, just observing that as well and gently bringing yourself back to the awareness of thinking. Letting go, beginning again each time you become involved in a thought. If you notice your mind repeatedly getting lost in thoughts you can always reconnect with the here and now by bringing your awareness back to the movements of the breath. Continuing to practice observing thoughts as they arise and pass for a few more moments.

Gently shifting your attention now from observing thoughts to an awareness of any emotions or feelings that are present. Maybe sadness, frustration, irritation. Or maybe joy or maybe boredom. Whatever you notice. Seeing if you can allow yourself to soften and open to any feelings that are here. What does this emotion feel like? Is it subtle or is it more pronounced? Where is it in the body? Maybe there are specific sensations that go with this emotion. Maybe there is tingling or tension somewhere. Maybe heaviness in the chest or perhaps the heartbeat speeds up. Maybe there is warmth or pressure somewhere. Or maybe it's just a general sense that permeates the whole body. Just see what you can notice. Acknowledging what's there and letting it be.

In these last few moments, seeing if you can hold the whole body in awareness: the breath falling in and out of the body, the other sensations throughout the body, any thoughts that arise.

This is a poem by Rumi called "The Guest House."

THE GUEST HOUSE

This being human is a guest house.
Every morning a new arrival.
A joy, a depression, a meanness,
Some momentary awareness comes
As an unexpected visitor.

Welcome and entertain them all!
Even if they're a crowd of sorrows,
Who violently* sweep your house
Empty of its furniture.

Still, treat each guest honorably.
He** may be clearing you out
For some new delight.

The dark thought, the shame, the malice.
Meet them at the door laughing,
And invite them in.

Be grateful for whoever comes,
Because each has been sent
As a guide from beyond.

As we shift now out of this practice, very gently allowing your awareness to expand to the presence of others in the room and the world around you.

Based on Segal, Williams, and Teasdale (2013). "The Guest House" is from Barks (1995). Copyright © 1995 Coleman Barks. Reprinted by permission.

*This word can be omitted.
**We suggest replacing "He" with "It" or "They."

SOBER Space (in Pairs)
PRACTICE 5.2

Intentions

+ Generalizing SOBER practice to everyday challenges by provoking a slightly more agitated, distracted, or "automatic" mode
+ Practicing mindful pausing in the context of an interpersonal exchange

---

We're going to practice the SOBER space, just as we did last week, but try it a little differently this time.

First, I'd like you to break into pairs. You'll have a discussion with the other person about something that frustrates or really annoys you. It could be something that happened today, maybe on your way over here—maybe someone cut you off in traffic or you spent a long time waiting for the bus. I encourage you to pick something fairly simple, not the greatest annoyance in your life. Does everyone have something in mind? Just talk with each other as you typically would during a break or before or after class—you don't have to take turns talking, in other words. Let it just be a conversation. We'll have you talk to each other for a few minutes, then when you hear the bell, stop wherever you are, even if in midsentence, and I'll give you some instructions.

(Allow talking in pairs for a minute or two or until it seems people are engrossed in the conversation, then ring the bell.)

Okay, wherever you are, just stop right here in this moment. Now shift your attention from your conversation to your internal experience, observing what is going on with you right now. What sensations are in the body? What feelings or emotions are present? What thoughts are going through your mind? Just noting the whole experience, without judging it or needing to change anything.

Now gathering awareness by focusing on the breath. By bringing attention to the rise and fall of the abdomen, or to the sensations of the breath moving in and out of the nostrils, and staying with those sensations for a few breaths.

And now allowing your awareness to expand, to include a sense of the body as a whole, all the sensations that are here, the quality of the mind and any thoughts, as well as any feelings or emotions.

And then finally, from this place of greater awareness, notice that you can make any one of a series of choices in how to respond. Maybe reflecting briefly on your interaction with your practice partner, and sensing if there is anything you might want to say or do differently. If you'd like to say anything to your partner, take a moment to do so now. If not, maybe just thank them and turn back into the circle.

Using the SOBER Space in Challenging Situations Worksheet
HANDOUT 5.1

Instructions: In the left column, list people, locations, relationships, emotions, or events that happen this week that feel challenging, triggering, or like high-risk situations for you. In the next columns, write what you notice about your reactions, specifically sensations, thoughts, or emotions that might be cues for you in the future to take a SOBER space. In the third column, note whether you were able to take a SOBER space, and in the final column, note how you responded in this situation.

High-risk situations or triggers (people, locations, emotions, events)	Reactions (sensations, thoughts, feelings that might be cues to take a SOBER space)	SOBER space? (yes/no)	How did you respond?

The reactions listed in the second column may be cues to stop and take a SOBER space. You may use these reactions as a reminder to step out of an automatic, reactive mode and observe your experience.

From *Mindfulness-Based Relapse Prevention for Addictive Behaviors, Second Edition: A Clinician's Guide* by Sarah Bowen, Neha Chawla, Joel Grow, and G. Alan Marlatt. Copyright © 2021 The Guilford Press. Permission to photocopy this handout is granted to purchasers of this book for personal use (see copyright page for details). Purchasers can download additional copies of this material (see the box at the end of the table of contents).

THEME

It can sometimes be challenging to accept what is arising in a particular situation. However, this is often the first step toward taking healthy or positive action in our lives. For example, we might not have control over things that happen to us, emotions that arise, our current job or family situation, or people's behaviors and reactions around us. When we fight against these things, however, we tend to feel frustrated, angry, or defeated, which can be triggers for substance use or other reactive behaviors. When we accept the present as it is, we are *not being passive*; we are allowing what already is without struggle or resistance. This is often a necessary and active first step toward change. The same is true of self-acceptance; it often requires a complete acceptance of ourselves as we are before real change can occur.

INTEGRATING PRACTICE INTO YOUR WEEK

1. Practice sitting meditation, body scan, or mindful movement. Note your practice on the Daily Practice Tracking Sheet (Handout 5.3).

2. Practice the SOBER space regularly and whenever you notice challenging emotions, sensations, or urges or anytime you notice yourself becoming reactive. Note your practice on the Daily Practice Tracking Sheet.

3. Complete the Using the SOBER Space in Challenging Situations Worksheet (Handout 5.1).

Daily Practice Tracking Sheet
HANDOUT 5.3

Instructions: Each day, record your mindfulness practice, also noting any barriers, observations, or comments.

Day/ date	Formal practice: How long?	SOBER space	Notes/comments
	____ minutes	How often? In what situations?	
	____ minutes	How often? In what situations?	
	____ minutes	How often? In what situations?	
	____ minutes	How often? In what situations?	
	____ minutes	How often? In what situations?	
	____ minutes	How often? In what situations?	
	____ minutes	How often? In what situations?	

SESSION 6

Seeing Thoughts as Thoughts

Our thoughts are just thoughts, not the truth of things, and
certainly not accurate representations of who we are. In being
seen and known, they cannot but self-liberate, and we are, in
that moment, liberated from them.

—Jon Kabat-Zinn

Materials

- Bell
- Whiteboard/markers
- Handout 6.1: Relapse Cycle Worksheet
- Handout 6.2: Session 6 Theme and Daily Practice: Seeing Thoughts as Thoughts
- Handout 6.3: Daily Practice Tracking Sheet
- Audio file: Sitting Meditation (Thoughts)

Theme

We have had a lot of practice over the past several weeks noticing our minds
wandering and labeling what is going on in the mind as "thinking." We have
practiced gently returning the focus of attention to the breath or body. Now we
want to turn our focus directly to thoughts and begin to relate to thoughts as
just words or images in the mind that we may or may not choose to believe or

engage in. We will discuss the role of thoughts, and believing our thoughts, in the relapse cycle.

Goals

- Reduce the degree of identification with thoughts and recognize that we don't have to buy into them or try to control them.
- Discuss the relapse cycle and the role of thoughts in perpetuating this cycle.

Session Outline

- Check-In
- Sitting Meditation: Thoughts (Practice 6.1)
- Daily Practice Review
- Thoughts and Relapse
- Relapse Cycle
- SOBER Space (Practice 6.2)
- Preparation for the End of the Course and Daily Practice
- Closing

Practice for This Week

- Practice using own selection
- SOBER space

CHECK-IN

In addition to the one- to two-word check-in, as practiced in the previous sessions, facilitators may begin with a moment of reflection, inviting participants to revisit their intentions for the course.

SITTING MEDITATION: THOUGHTS

At this stage in the course, participants have had the experience of using the breath as a primary anchor for their attention and gradually expanding awareness to include sounds, sensations, and mental and emotional experiences. Although they have been encouraged throughout the course to become aware of thoughts and the relationships between thoughts, emotions, and sensations, focus on mental activity is made more explicit in this session (Practice 6.1). Participants are asked to practice allowing thoughts to be the primary object of their awareness, stepping back from their content and observing the nature of thinking itself.

In the current session, we begin by observing the presence of "thinking," then practice labeling different categories of thoughts that arise. Participants may begin to realize that thoughts are simply words or images arising in the mind rather than reliable reflections of the "truth." We then use metaphors to practice observing thoughts as they arise and watching as they pass. When we are aware we have become caught up in their content, we practice gently disentangling our attention and returning to observing their arising and passing. Like sounds or sensations, we can learn to observe them as they arise and pass, while staying in contact with the present moment.

Observing and Labeling Thoughts

In this session's practices, participants start by simply observing thoughts arising and passing, seeing if they can notice when a thought appears and when it naturally passes. They then move to a practice of labeling thoughts (e.g., "memory," "fantasy," "analyzing," "planning"). Then they are introduced to metaphors and imagery to aid in the practice of bringing awareness to the arising and passing of thoughts in the mind. For instance, they may imagine observing thoughts as leaves floating by on a stream or clouds moving across a clear sky. They are encouraged to experiment with labeling thoughts to increase recognition of thoughts as passing objects. This practice not only helps to step back from the content of thoughts but allows greater understanding of the various forms thoughts can take.

Following these practices, participants share their experiences of the metaphors and labeling as means of observing thoughts. We also suggest other metaphors, including thoughts as images or words on a movie screen or balloons floating away, and ask participants to be creative in generating metaphors that seem particularly relevant or useful for them. If participants note that their minds are particularly busy, we might suggest metaphors such as listening to a radio broadcast or to a tiny creature on one's shoulder delivering a running commentary; although it may not be possible to turn off the radio or silence the creature, it may be helpful to realize that it is simply a chattering voice and we have a choice in how we relate to it. If metaphors become complicated or distracting, they can be abandoned. The point is to practice relating to thoughts as arising and passing objects in the mind and learn to observe them versus getting involved in them. Sometimes metaphors can help with this practice.

The labeling practice may also be useful for some in creating distance and perspective. However, for others who do not find it useful or for whom it is a struggle, it need not be continued. Some participants report struggling to find the right label or getting caught up in the labeling itself. The purpose of the exercise is not to focus on the accuracy of the labels but to recognize arising thoughts and the tendency to become involved in them. If finding the "right" label becomes a struggle, a simple label of "thinking" can also be applied.

Often participants will report self-judgment as soon as they become aware of having been caught in a thought or story. This is an opportunity to recognize judgment as yet another thought. Participants are then encouraged to simply note "judging" rather than to try to get rid of judgment, which often just compounds it.

If participants report repeatedly getting lost in the content of a particular thought, they are encouraged to simply return their attention to the breath as a means of stabilizing the mind. Recurring thoughts or themes may reflect a feeling or emotion that one hasn't fully acknowledged or allowed into awareness. If the same thought continues to repeat itself, bringing attention to the feeling state or emotion behind the thought, noticing how it is experienced in the body and mind, can sometimes loosen its grip and power.

On occasion and with continued practice, the mind may be still enough to notice the beginning and end of thoughts and their ephemeral quality, but this recognition usually takes time and practice. The mind may get caught up in a story for several minutes or even hours before we become aware that we are no longer present. It is unreasonable to expect that our minds will suddenly behave exactly as we tell them to after we have let them run free for so many years. Thus, every moment of awareness and recognition that occurs between these wanderings is a moment of mindfulness and wakefulness; we are simply working to bring into our practice, and into our lives, more of these moments.

DAILY PRACTICE REVIEW

In the previous session, participants were given the option of practicing mindful movement in addition or as an alternative to the body scan and sitting meditation practices. Exploring the varied responses to the movement practice is a valuable part of this session's daily practice review. Several participants have reported enjoying the opportunity to engage in the practice and relating to their bodies with greater gentleness and caring. This may be particularly helpful for those experiencing significant physical discomfort, stiffness, or pain. Again, it is important to emphasize that the purpose is not to push the body or engage in postures that may be painful but to become aware of the body in movement and to bring care and compassion to experiences of pleasure or discomfort.

Participants sometimes report that the movement practice is easier or more enjoyable than the sitting meditation. In such cases, it is helpful to explore what aspects of the practice are enjoyable as well as those that may be challenging when practicing sitting. Participants may feel that it is easier to be "doing something" rather than simply paying attention to their mental states. In this case, we typically encourage participants to experience each of the different practices with openness and reiterate that experiences of discomfort, restlessness, or self-judgment that arise are all part of mindfulness practice, allowing valuable opportunities for further observation of the mind.

In the previous session, participants were also asked to continue incorporating the SOBER space and to note situations in which they used this practice, what they observed, and how they responded in the situation. In discussing these experiences, an effort is made to help participants identify specific cues in each of those situations that might be future reminders for practicing SOBER space (e.g., shoulders and jaw becoming tense, feeling anger arising, blaming and judging thoughts about one's spouse, having the thought "I can't take this anymore"). Reviewing these aloud can help participants remember them as personal cues for engaging in SOBER or another mindfulness practice.

THOUGHTS AND RELAPSE

The previous discussion often flows naturally into a conversation about the role of thoughts in the relapse process. We ask participants to define thoughts, asking whether or not thoughts are "true." This typically leads to the recognition that thoughts are simply ideas, memories, images, and strings of words that arise in the mind from moment to moment that may or may not be reflective of reality. Although some are easy to let go of, others have a more enticing or "sticky" quality.

Participants are often quick to recognize the automaticity of thinking and the link between thoughts and behavior. They typically point out that there is a choice in whether or not to believe, follow, or act upon thoughts. Occasionally, participants have trouble with the idea that thoughts are not always reliable reflections of reality. We have found it helpful to use metaphors and examples to illustrate that thoughts are simply words and images arising in the mind. For example, one might imagine being caught up in the story line of a movie and having the sudden recognition that one is actually an observer sitting in the audience, that it is only a story. Or one might imagine the mind continually creating thoughts and stories like the heart pumping blood or the stomach secreting bile; it is simply another organ in the body, and producing thoughts and stories is its job. The stories it produces, however, may or may not be grounded in reality. Examples of specific thoughts to which one has held strongly in the past that turned out not to be true can also illustrate how thoughts are not always trustworthy.

RELAPSE CYCLE

To further illustrate the relationship between thoughts and relapse, participants are asked to provide an example of an event that has been or may potentially be a trigger, either for substance use or relapse, or for another reactive, cyclical behavior in their lives. Typically, we choose one example from the group to walk through, illustrating it on the board following the basic template of the relapse cycle (see Figure 6.1) and showing the possible paths that different choices might lead to.

Participants are asked to break down the chain of events by identifying initial thoughts, feelings, and physical reactions that may have arisen in their minds when encountering the triggering situation as well as any emotional reactions or sensations they may have experienced. They are then asked to follow the situation through to the point of lapse or full-blown relapse or, alternatively, to points in the cycle at which they may have stepped back and responded differently (Handout 6.1), using practices learned thus far to step out of "automatic pilot" and make more conscious, kind choices at any point along the way. The form that this discussion takes seems to vary from group to group, depending on the unique histories

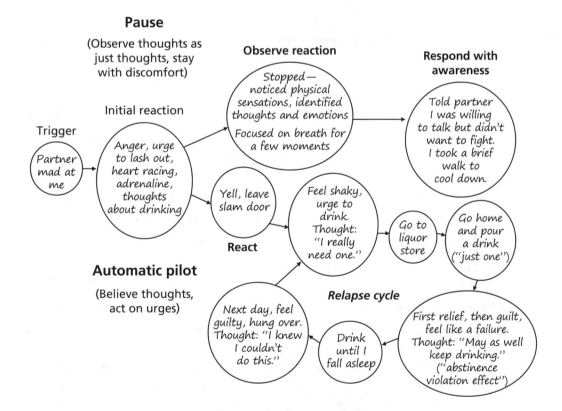

FIGURE 6.1. Relapse cycle.

and perspectives of the participants. We have found it most useful to be open to this variability while keeping at the core of the discussion the notion that thoughts play a powerful role at each point in the relapse cycle, and that slowing down and observing one's thoughts, emotional states, and physical reactions can create an opportunity to step out of the cycle and choose a more skillful response. The following is one example of this discussion:

> FACILITATOR: Okay, is someone willing to offer an example of a situation that has led to a relapse or another reactive behavior in the past, or that you imagine could put you at risk in the future?
>
> PARTICIPANT 1: I will. When I get into a fight with my wife, depending on how bad it is, it may lead me to want to drink.
>
> FACILITATOR: Okay, let's just stay with this example and walk through it if that's okay with you? So the initial trigger is a fight with your wife. What kind of thoughts might come into your mind when that happens?
>
> PARTICIPANT 1: Well, I would be angry.
>
> FACILITATOR: So there is an emotional reaction, and maybe some physical sensations, too? (*Makes notes on whiteboard.*)
>
> PARTICIPANT 1: Yeah, heart racing and blood pressure rising.
>
> FACILITATOR: And what thoughts might you have when you feel this way?
>
> PARTICIPANT 1: Generally, for me it's a "screw it" sort of attitude that leads me to pick up again.
>
> FACILITATOR: So let's break that down. What's a specific thought that might go through your mind?
>
> PARTICIPANT 1: "Screw it, I have been trying really hard and it just doesn't seem to work."
>
> FACILITATOR: Okay. (*Notes this on board.*) What happens next?
>
> PARTICIPANT 1: I leave the house and head to the liquor store.
>
> FACILITATOR: Does that feel "automatic" or more thoughtful or aware?
>
> PARTICIPANT 1: Automatic, definitely. I don't stop and observe. It's totally autopilot.
>
> FACILITATOR: Okay. So there's this trigger, then this series of reactions in your body and mind and emotions, that can lead, if you are on autopilot, to a behavior—in this case, drinking.
>
> Is there ever a time when this has gone differently? Or can you imagine it going differently? Let's imagine you have the same fight with your wife and the same emotion and the thought, even, of "Screw it, it's not

working." Up to that point, maybe none of what has arisen is really in your control—the raw emotion, the physical sensations, and even the thought "screw it." These reactions often just arise when we are triggered; it's what our bodies and minds do and we may or may not be able to change that, at least for now. But we do have a choice in where to go from there. Say at that moment you notice that reaction or that thought, you recognize it, and you stop for a moment to observe what's happening rather than just reacting in your habitual way. What might happen then?

PARTICIPANT 1: I think that would be a powerful way of interrupting this process.

FACILITATOR: What do you think might happen if you stopped and just noticed what you were experiencing?

PARTICIPANT 1: I might realize that my reaction is not necessary; it's irrational. And maybe I would think about the consequences of my actions.

FACILITATOR: Okay, so first of all there is some awareness of what is going on for you—the anger and thoughts of wanting to drink. And you used the word "irrational." Maybe by stopping and noticing how your mind and body are reacting, you aren't believing those thoughts quite as much. Here's this thought, "Screw it, it's not working," and maybe you recognize this as only a thought and notice, too, that you don't have to act on it.

PARTICIPANT 1: If I could stop in that moment, I would have the recognition that it's not true, and I would see that I don't have to go there.

FACILITATOR: So it seems like for you, stopping immediately provides the opportunity to step back and recognize that you don't have to take that route, that you don't have to buy into what your mind and body are telling you to do. So once you stop, what would you do next?

PARTICIPANT 1: Well, I think I would think about the consequences of my actions and I wouldn't recklessly act on my thought and emotion. I wouldn't leave the house and get in the car to head to the liquor store. Maybe I would go upstairs and be by myself for awhile, or tell my wife I really didn't want to fight anymore.

FACILITATOR: A really different response than the first one.

PARTICIPANT 1: I have gone both ways in this scenario. I've gone to drink, and I've stopped and disengaged from that slippery slope.

FACILITATOR: Okay, then let's follow the other route for a second. Say you do have that thought "Screw it, not worth it" and you buy into it and drive to the liquor store. What then?

The discussion then follows an example of events and experiences that led up to a lapse, and it continues past that lapse to illustrate that, following a lapse, there is still some choice; things don't have to continue to cycle downwards. Some participants feel strongly that after the initial choice of whether to believe the thoughts or after they have behaved reactively to a trigger, they no longer have a choice; it is too late. However, others might consider that the moment of the first drink or use presents another choice point where they can continue along that path or stop and turn around. Our approach to this discussion has been to make room for all of these reactions and experiences while helping participants break down this seemingly automatic process, step by step, suggesting that thoughts following initial substance use (e.g., "I blew it, it's over") are thoughts as well.

The intense self-judgment that often occurs following an initial lapse, referred to as the "abstinence violation effect" (Marlatt & Donovan, 2005), may increase the likelihood of experiencing a full-blown relapse. This discussion can serve as preparation, highlighting the possibility of minimizing the potential damage resulting from a lapse, were it to occur. This discussion also reflects a mindful and accepting stance, encouraging honesty and openness in the face of difficulty. The following is a continuation of the previous dialogue:

PARTICIPANT 1: That's a relapse for me. At that point I am in that spiral, and I am not thinking of anything. I'm just on a mission. It's too late.

PARTICIPANT 2: Yeah, me too. If I allow my mind to go from the trigger to following the thought, I am already in trouble. If I don't separate my thoughts at that point, I am a done deal. I am going to end up homeless or in jail and it's all over.

FACILITATOR: So for both of you this is a really crucial point. So it's important to do everything you can to be aware of the direction you're heading in before you end up using. What if we follow this a little further and see what happens? Is it all right if we do that? In the past, when you have gotten to the point of using and spiraled so quickly, is there anything you can think of that might have helped you turn around a little sooner? That might have prevented you from going down that path until you ended up homeless or in jail?

[Facilitator and participant review the thoughts and actions in this familiar scenario, pausing at each step to recognize what thoughts might have been arising, whether or not those thoughts were "trustworthy" or "true," and the effects of believing those thoughts. The facilitator also inquires about all the cues the participant might notice in the future for taking a SOBER space and stepping out of the cycle, even when his mind was telling him it was "too late."]

FACILITATOR: It's going to be a different process for each person. What's important is that you get to know how your mind works, and points at which you've gotten in trouble in the past where maybe you could do something differently if that were to come up again. What we are doing here is highlighting different points at which you may have a choice and can shift the course. So, in this example, when you get to this point here (where you have had the first drink), what goes through your mind?

PARTICIPANT 3: I've already screwed up.

FACILITATOR: Right, "I've already screwed up, why stop now? I might as well go all the way."

PARTICIPANT 3: Exactly.

FACILITATOR: And even though you are already in trouble at this point, does it have to be all over? That thought, "I've already screwed up," even though it is an extremely powerful and consuming thought, it is still a thought. I don't want to minimize the dangerousness and seriousness of the situation, but if you do end up in this very dangerous place, does it have to be "a done deal"?

PARTICIPANT 3: No. Maybe it's possible to at least minimize the damage.

FACILITATOR: So what do you all make of this? Thoughts or reactions as you look at this up on the board?

SOBER SPACE

Given that participants often have strong reactions to this conversation, it can be helpful to conclude with a SOBER space (Practice 6.2) as an opportunity to observe one's reactions, thoughts, and emotions and to reconnect with the present. The SOBER space in this session might emphasize awareness of arising thoughts.

PREPARATION FOR THE END OF THE COURSE AND DAILY PRACTICE

At this stage in the program, participants are encouraged to begin exploring ways to personalize the practice and make it a part of their daily lives. In this spirit, they are encouraged to choose a selection of practices from the options offered in previous weeks (Handout 6.2). It can be helpful to provide additional audio recordings of shorter practices of 10, 20, and 30 minutes, or practices without verbal instructions (i.e., just the sound of a bell as a reminder to return awareness to the present). Although participants may experiment with combinations of these practices, they are encouraged to continue with some sort of practice each day to maintain and continue to build on the skills gained during the course. In preparation for continuing practice following the course, participants are asked to begin reflecting on what they have learned over the past several weeks and which practices they intend to continue. It is suggested that they continue integrating the SOBER space into their daily lives, particularly in situations in which they feel overwhelmed or reactive. Participants are also asked to record their practice on the Daily Practice Tracking Sheet (Handout 6.3).

CLOSING

Facilitators may choose to close with a moment of silence and/or a brief checkout.

Sitting Meditation
Thoughts
PRACTICE 6.1

Intentions

+ Observing thoughts similarly to how we have been observing sounds and sensation—as arising and passing objects of attention

+ Creating distance and perspective by observing thoughts as objects while stepping back from their content, using metaphors to observe the arising and passing of thoughts in the mind

+ Viewing thoughts as simply words or images arising in the mind, rather than reliable reflections of truth

+ Recognizing a judgment as yet another thought

PART I

This is a brief practice in which we see what it's like to watch our own minds. So we'll just spend a few minutes observing what is happening in our mind—specifically watching thoughts as they come and go. Let's do this by either closing our eyes or resting the eyes on a spot on the floor. The instruction is to watch your mind—and when you notice a thought arise, you can raise your hand. When the thought passes, you can put your hand down. If two thoughts come at once, maybe you raise both hands. Questions? Okay—begin when you are ready. (Allow 1–2 minutes.)

What was that like? (brief inquiry)

What are thoughts, anyway? (write ideas on the board)

What are some different categories of thoughts? (write sample categories on the board, such as memories, fantasies, planning, images, judgments)

PART II

Okay, we'll do a similar exercise now, but we'll try labeling the thoughts that arise, using these categories on the board, or maybe other ones that fit. So as each thought comes up, see if you can recognize the type of thought, apply a label, then let it go. If you're not sure what category a thought falls into, don't worry about it—you can just label it "thought" and let it pass. No need to raise hands on this one. Any questions? Okay, begin when you're ready. (Allow 1–2 minutes.)

Okay, what was that like? What did you notice?

PART III

Okay, for this last practice, we'll bring these practices together. Begin by settling in your chair, closing your eyes if you choose to. Sitting with a calm, dignified, and wakeful presence, with your spine upright and body relaxed. Taking a moment to become aware of yourself here in this room at this moment. Bringing awareness to your body here in the chair.

Now gathering the attention and bringing it to your breath: the inbreath, the outbreath, the waves of breath as they enter and leave your body. Not looking for anything

(continued)

to happen or for any special state or experience, just continuing to stay with the sensations of breathing for the next few moments.

Now letting the breath fade into the background of your attention, allowing your awareness to focus on the thoughts that are arising in your mind. See if you can notice the very next thought, then let it naturally pass, and then see if you can notice the next thought, allowing that to pass by, too, without becoming involved in it or following it.

As we practice this, I am going suggest a metaphor that you can try if it is useful. If not, modify it however you'd like or drop it altogether. You might imagine that you are sitting by a stream. Take a moment now to picture this stream in your mind. It might be a familiar stream, or you can just make one up. Now, as thoughts begin to arise, imagine you are sitting on the shore watching them float by as though they were leaves on the water. As you become aware of each thought that appears, just gently allow it to float by, just like leaves on a stream. The thoughts might be words or an image or a sentence. Some thoughts might be larger or heavier, some smaller, quicker, or lighter. Whatever form the thought is in, as the next one appears, do the same, allowing it to float by. Just doing your best with this. If you find that you are worrying about what it should look like or whether you are doing this right, just notice that these, too, are thoughts on the passing stream. If thoughts come quickly, you might picture the stream rushing with white water. As the thoughts calm down, the stream might slow down and flow more smoothly.

If you find that you become lost in a thought or your attention has been carried downstream by a thought, you might congratulate yourself for becoming aware again, noticing, if possible, what thought pulled you away and then simply step back out of the stream and resume sitting on the bank, observing passing thoughts.

Something you might try here is labeling thoughts as they appear. Maybe they are judgments about yourself, your experience, or how you are doing on this exercise. If so, just label that thought as "judgment" and let it pass. Perhaps you have a memory arise. If so, you might just label it as "memory." Or perhaps plans come to mind about what you are going to do after today's session or what you are going to say to someone in the future. Often fantasies come to mind. We imagine scenarios that might happen or that we would like to happen. Just recognize the thoughts as judgments, memories, plans, fantasies, or any labels that work for you, and allow the thoughts to pass. Try practicing this now. If no labels come to mind, that's okay, too. You might just use the label "thought" or simply notice that no labels come to mind and continue to observe.

If you find you are lost in one of the thoughts that has arisen, notice what that thought was that carried you away, then gently bring yourself back to the exercise of observing.

Now, very gently and when you are ready, allowing your awareness to focus on the room here, your body in this chair, awareness of the other people here with you in the room. Giving yourself time to very gently allow your eyes to open, if they are closed. Holding this awareness, as best you can, as your eyes take in the room and the people around you.

SOBER Space

Let's take a moment to pause here. Begin by observing, becoming aware of what is going on with you right now—what sensations do you notice? Are there thoughts? What are you saying to yourself? What is the quality of your mind right now? Is it calm? Agitated? Rushing with thoughts? Quiet? And finally, any emotions you can detect?

Now gathering your awareness and bringing it to the breath . . . the movements of the abdomen, the rise and fall of the breath, moment by moment, each inhale and exhale.

Now allowing your awareness to expand to include a sense of the body as a whole. Holding your entire body in this slightly softer, more spacious awareness, noticing again what sensations are here, what thoughts are present, the quality of the mind, and any moods or emotions. Notice that you have many choices in how you move forward from here.

Relapse Cycle Worksheet
HANDOUT 6.1

Think of a situation that has led to a reactive behavior in the past, or a situation you imagine might be risky for you in the future. Write the trigger, the initial reaction that followed, and the events along each possible path in the circles below. *How might your responses differ if you are on autopilot versus if you are more aware?*

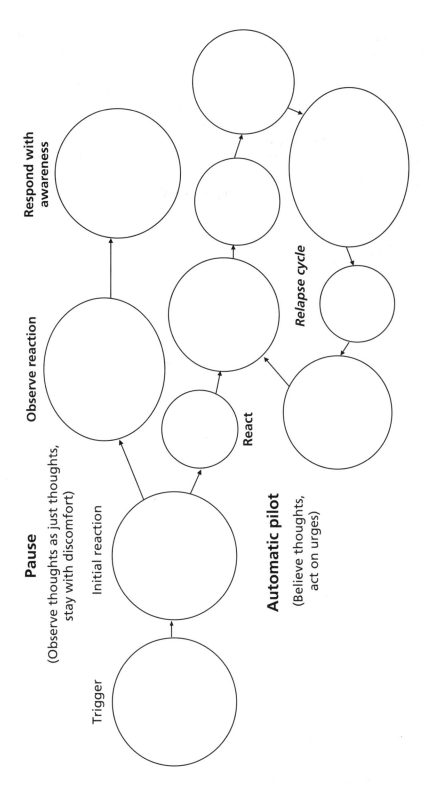

Respond with awareness

Observe reaction

Pause
(Observe thoughts as just thoughts, stay with discomfort)

Initial reaction

Trigger

React

Relapse cycle

Automatic pilot
(Believe thoughts, act on urges)

Seeing Thoughts as Thoughts
HANDOUT 6.2

THEME

We have had a lot of practice noticing our minds wandering. We have practiced gently returning the focus of attention to the breath or body sensations. Now we want to intentionally turn our focus to thoughts and practice relating to them as just words or images in the mind that we may or may not choose to believe. In this session, we discuss the role of thoughts in the relapse process and, more specifically, what tends to happen when we believe these thoughts.

INTEGRATING PRACTICE INTO YOUR WEEK

1. Choose your own practice from the set of practices we've learned thus far. Note your practice on the Daily Practice Tracking Sheet.

2. Practice the SOBER space regularly and whenever you notice challenging emotions, sensations, and urges or anytime you notice yourself becoming reactive. Note your practice on the Daily Practice Tracking Sheet.

3. Complete the Relapse Cycle Worksheet.

Instructions: Each day, record your mindfulness practice, also noting any barriers, observations, or comments.

Day/ date	Formal practice with audio recording: How long?	SOBER space	Notes/comments
	____ minutes	How often? In what situations?	
	____ minutes	How often? In what situations?	
	____ minutes	How often? In what situations?	
	____ minutes	How often? In what situations?	
	____ minutes	How often? In what situations?	
	____ minutes	How often? In what situations?	
	____ minutes	How often? In what situations?	

Supporting and Sustaining Well-Being

This is why we practice meditation—so that we can treat ourselves more compassionately; improve our relationships with friends, family, and community; live lives of greater connection; and, even in the face of challenges, stay in touch with what we really care about so we can act in ways that are consistent with our values.

—SHARON SALZBERG

Materials

- Bell
- Whiteboard/markers
- Handout 7.1: Daily Activities Worksheet
- Handout 7.2: Reminder Card
- Handout 7.3: Session 7 Theme and Daily Practice: Supporting and Sustaining Well-Being
- Handout 7.4: Daily Practice Tracking Sheet
- Audio file: Kindness Meditation

Theme

We have spent several weeks paying close attention to the specific situations, thoughts, and emotions that put us at risk for relapse. In this session, we take a look at the broader picture of our lives and identify those aspects that support a healthier, more vital life and those that put us at greater risk. Taking care of oneself and engaging in nourishing activities are an essential part of recovery.

Goals

- Discuss the importance of lifestyle balance and self-care in reducing vulnerability to relapse.
- Discuss the use of regular mindfulness practice as a means of maintaining overall well-being.
- Prepare for future high-risk situations using the Reminder Card.

Session Outline

- Check-In
- Kindness Meditation (Practice 7.1)
- Practice Review
- Daily Activities Worksheet
- Where Does Relapse Begin?
- SOBER Space
- Reminder Cards
- Daily Practice
- Closing

Practice for This Week

- Practice using own selection
- SOBER space

CHECK-IN

In these final sessions, it is useful to begin with a reflection on what elements of the course participants have found to be most valuable and what they intend to continue practicing in their daily lives. The check-in in this session can provide an opportunity for participants to recall and recommit to this intention.

KINDNESS MEDITATION

This session introduces a sitting meditation that focuses on what is traditionally called lovingkindness—friendliness, goodwill, or compassion (Practice 7.1).

Depending on the group, this can simply be called kindness practice, if participants are uncomfortable with the term "lovingkindness." Traditionally, kindness, or lovingkindness, practice involves bringing attention to a set of well-wishes such as *May I be safe and free from harm, May I be peaceful, and May I live with ease.* Individuals may modify these well-wishes as needed and use visualization if helpful. We encourage facilitators to explore these practices in their groups if it feels comfortable and appropriate, and to be creative in choosing instructions that seem most genuine, appropriate, and relevant for their participants.

Practicing kindness sometimes gives rise to feelings of resistance or aversion, or other challenging experiences. Participants may comment that it "didn't work," alluding to a failure to feel kindness toward themselves or others. However, as with all the practices thus far, observing these reactions and difficulties with a kind, nonjudgmental attitude is as much a part of the practice as feelings of well-being, openness, and ease. We have found it useful to address this and remind participants that there is no "right" experience. *Kindness practice is not intended to bring about a certain feeling or mind state, but rather involves observing whatever arises as we practice.*

PRACTICE REVIEW

Over the previous week, participants were instructed to engage in their own patterns of practice. As part of the practice review, we invite participants to share what they are noticing in the process of making the practice "their own," indicate whether they have been able to find a routine that feels sustainable, and address ongoing barriers and challenges. Participants have also been continuing their practice of the SOBER space and may have experiences to share. Finally, sharing a few examples from the Relapse Cycle Worksheet (Handout 6.1), which clients were asked to complete during the previous week, helps reiterate the importance of "stepping out" of the relapse process as early as possible and sets the stage for Session 7, in which we widen the focus to a broader picture of relapse risks and lifestyle balance.

DAILY ACTIVITIES WORKSHEET

The Daily Activities Worksheet (Handout 7.1), an adaptation of exercises from MBCT (Segal et al., 2013) and from Daley and Marlatt's (2006) relapse prevention protocol, is a tool intended to bring awareness to typical daily activities and how they tend to affect overall mood, life balance, and health, discussed below in terms of "nourishing" and "depleting" effects. This exercise encourages reflection on the manner in which we engage in these activities and whether there are ways we tend to make a "neutral" activity depleting or a neutral or depleting activity more nourishing. It is an opportunity to have participants notice the actual qualities of each experience and to differentiate those from additional "layers" or "add-ons" they may be adding that make it more depleting.

In the first part of this exercise, using the Daily Activities Worksheet, participants compile lists of activities, people, and situations in their lives that feel depleting (e.g., discouraging, exhausting, frustrating, draining) and that feel nourishing (e.g., energizing, pleasurable, rejuvenating, satisfying). Participants then describe how they tend to feel during or after the activity.

Inquiry might begin with an open question about what people notice. It can be interesting to ask people to look at the right-hand column—the qualities these things elicit. It may be informative to see what feelings or reactions we have that are, for each of us, nourishing or depleting.

In the next part of this exercise, participants list activities of a typical day on the back of the worksheet. Then they are instructed to review their list and identify each activity as either nourishing ("N") or depleting ("D"). Participants then look at the balance between the "N"s and the "D"s.

Again, inquiry can begin with an open-ended question about what people noticed. Participants are often surprised by having either more nourishing activities or more depleting activities in their day than they anticipated. They often remark on how the same activity may be nourishing or depleting, depending on their state of mind, other factors in their lives, or the way in which they approach it. This exercise not only offers perspective on how we spend our days and the balance between depleting versus nourishing activities, but also elicits discussion of the importance of including more nourishing activities or engaging in activities in a way that might be less depleting.

The purpose of this exercise is not to encourage participants to eradicate all depleting activities (although the addition of more daily activities that feed us in a healthful way, even seemingly small ones, certainly has benefits to our mood and functioning). Rather, it is intended to bring greater awareness to how we spend our days, the quality of attention and presence we bring to our activities, and how both the activities and our quality of attention to them tend to affect us. Some depleting or stressful activities might be avoidable; others may not. This is an opportunity to notice what is nourishing and depleting, and to explore how we might relate to experiences differently. Further, discussion can also include how mindfulness practice helps this process and how the ways we relate to daily activities might increase risk for relapse.

Following the inquiry for Part 2, we then ask participants to choose one thing on their list that is nourishing and that they might sometimes "miss" because their attention is elsewhere. For example, perhaps while showering, which can be a pleasurable activity, the mind is already planning the day or reworking something that happened yesterday. Other examples might be drinking coffee or tea in the morning, putting on pajamas at night, or walking a dog. We invite participants to close their eyes for a few moments and imagine engaging in this activity, noticing its qualities.

> FACILITATOR: What are the things that make it enjoyable or nourishing? Are there sensations? See if you can feel those now. How about sounds? Smells? Tastes? Or maybe a quality of mind or a general feeling this activity brings you. Take a moment to imagine this and come into contact as best you can with these qualities, seeing if you might allow them fully rather than rushing through them. By bringing awareness to this activity, we are in more direct contact with its inherently nourishing qualities, such as the feel of warm water or sudsy shampoo. We can get more nourishment from this activity simply by bringing attention to it as we engage in it.

We then suggest participants experiment with bringing this kind of presence and attention to a few things in the upcoming week that might actually be nourishing or enjoyable.

Daily practice for this session includes choosing at least three activities that are nourishing and engaging in them over the upcoming week. It is important that participants choose activities that are realistic and to which they can commit. These can either be new activities or ones in which they already engage. It can be helpful to have participants state aloud what activities they are committing to as a way to remember to do them.

WHERE DOES RELAPSE BEGIN?

Until now, discussions and exercises have focused largely on proximal triggers for relapse (e.g., people, places, thoughts, emotions). This session begins to widen the focus to lifestyle choices that make us more or less vulnerable to these triggers.

For example, imagine that a participant is walking down a street and sees someone with whom she used to drink. On a particular day, she may be able to handle this situation skillfully, choosing to turn the corner and take a different route or say hello and tell her friend she is no longer drinking, then continue walking. On another day, she might encounter this same friend and choose to engage in conversation, not mention to her friend that she is in recovery, accept the friend's invitation to go to their favorite bar to see some old friends, and then end up with a drink. In reviewing factors that may affect one's vulnerability in this situation, we elicit examples from the group, such as general stress level, exhaustion, loneliness, and lack of social support. We often mention the acronym HALT (*H*ungry, *A*ngry, *L*onely, *T*ired) from the 12-step tradition as an example of factors influencing vulnerability. In this exercise, it is helpful to highlight that these are common experiences that will continue to arise in our lives. Recognizing them as warning signs can remind us to take better care of ourselves and alert us to our increased vulnerability to triggers during these times. We might check in when feeling triggered ("Am I hungry? Sad? Lonely? Anxious?") as a way to understand our reaction to a trigger and to identify what we need to do to best take care of ourselves ("What is it I really need right now?").

SOBER SPACE

Often after discussions, especially those that are more conceptual or that elicit some reaction, facilitators might suggest pausing with a SOBER space. It can be helpful to practice these in different ways throughout the course. For example, facilitators might suggest trying the exercise with eyes open and might vary the length of time spent engaged in the exercise. These variations can help increase flexibility and generalizability of this practice.

REMINDER CARDS

The Reminder Card (Handout 7.2) is intended as a reminder of each individual's available skills and support. About the size of a business card, it has four quadrants (two on each side of a folded piece of paper). They contain participants' personalized list of reasons to stay on track, alternative activities/plans, resources, and the steps of the SOBER space. The Reminder Card is designed to fit easily in a pocket or wallet, readily accessible as a reminder and for use in high-risk situations.

While the card itself may be dated due to advances in technology, the reflections involved in the exercise are still likely to be useful. One possibility would be to have participants write down their responses and take a photo to save as the background image on their phones, if they feel so inclined.

Ideally, the Reminder Card is discussed and completed in session because participants can benefit from others' thoughts and ideas. For example, some participants might share a significant reason for maintaining treatment goals that is particularly powerful or salient for others and thus important to include on the card.

We often facilitate this exercise in four parts, drawing a horizontal and a vertical line on the board to separate the quadrants:

Quadrant 1: Reasons to stay on track. We ask people to reflect on what they've lost as a consequence of use or other behaviors, and which of these things might remind them of reasons to stay the course when things are challenging. [Write this on the board in Quadrant 1.]

Quadrant 2: Alternative activities/plans. In generating these, a facilitator might ask, "What are some things that you have done or might do to help when urges or cravings arise? Sometimes when we are reactive we lose sight of all the options we have, and it can be helpful to list these here when we have more clarity."

Quadrant 3: The SOBER space—a way to access alternative behaviors. We briefly review the steps of the SOBER practice noted on the card.

Quadrant 4: Resources. This section lists people whom participants can call, or where they might go for help or support. This quadrant of the card might contain preprinted names and/or phone numbers of local community resources and help lines, and participants are instructed to supplement this with contact information for their own personal resources or support systems. The Reminder Card should be completed with this additional information before the next session.

DAILY PRACTICE

For the upcoming week, we continue to encourage group members to create their own practice routine, choosing practices they intend to use on a regular basis. We also suggest continued practice of the SOBER space, both during routine daily activities and in higher-stress situations. Finally, we review the plan to engage in three specific nourishing activities (Handout 7.3) and instruct participants to complete the Reminder Card if there are additional ideas or resources they would like to add. Participants are also instructed to record meditation practice on the Daily Practice Tracking Sheet (Handout 7.4).

CLOSING

The last few moments of the session can provide another opportunity to have participants recall and reconnect with the practice intentions they identified at the beginning of the session, then close with a one- to two-word checkout.

Kindness Meditation
PRACTICE 7.1

Intentions

✦ Practicing kindness toward self and others

✦ Observing whatever arises in the practice (including resistance and aversion) with openness and curiosity, rather than expecting a particular feeling or sentiment

---

This meditation is slightly different from those we have practiced in the course thus far. It is a "friendliness" or kindness practice that involves developing a kinder, gentler attitude toward ourselves and others. This kind and compassionate approach is an important aspect of mindfulness practice and can help support the other practices that we have done.

As with other practices, it's important to remember that there is no special way you are supposed to feel. We're not trying to make ourselves suddenly feel differently toward ourselves and others. What we are doing is noticing what happens as we engage in this practice. So whatever comes up for you is fine—see if you can be aware of it and curious about it.

To begin, find a position that is comfortable for you, allowing your body to be at ease and just loosening any tension you might notice in your body. Allowing any tightness to release, softening your belly, gently releasing any tension in your arms and shoulders, your face, relaxing your jaw. Maybe taking a moment to connect with your intention, your reason for being here and engaging in this practice.

Feeling your body against the floor or the chair. Feeling the solidity and stability of the ground beneath you, allowing your body to release into the chair or the ground, and feeling a sense of safety here in this moment, allowing the ground to support you.

Now bring to mind someone you know personally, or know of, toward whom you naturally have feelings of friendliness and caring. It is best not to pick someone with whom you've had conflict or are romantically involved, but rather someone toward whom you feel an easy warmth and friendliness. It may be a friend or a relative, maybe a grandchild or grandparent. Or it could be a spiritual guide, or even a pet. Maybe someone who makes you naturally smile just thinking about them.

If you'd like, imagine that this someone is sitting next to you, by your side, or in front of you. If you are unable to picture this person or being, just allow yourself to focus on the feeling, the sensations you may experience in the presence of this being. Take a few minutes to pay attention to how you feel, sensing where in your body you experience feelings of compassion and caring. This may be in the center of your chest, where your heart is, or in the belly or the face. Wherever you feel the experience of caring or kindness in your body, with each breath, allow this area to soften. If you have trouble sensing this or finding the area where these feelings might be centered, it's okay. Just keep your focus on this general area of your heart and notice what, if anything, you can sense there throughout this exercise.

Now, if it feels comfortable to you, send this person or being well-wishes. We often use the following phrases, repeating them quietly in our minds:

May you be safe and protected. May you find true happiness. May you be peaceful. May you live with a sense of ease. (Repeat slowly.)

You can use these well-wishes or you can create your own, whatever feels most

(continued)

152

genuine for you. Continuing to repeat them mentally. *May you be safe and protected. May you be happy. May you be peaceful. May you live with a sense of ease.* Or whatever well-wishes you have chosen.

Again, the idea is not to make anything happen; we are simply sending well-wishes, the way you might wish someone a safe journey or a good day. If you find yourself having thoughts such as "This isn't working" or "This is silly," just noticing these thoughts and gently guiding your attention back to the wishes. Similarly, if you find yourself feeling frustrated or irritated, just bringing your attention to that experience, and remembering that you can always bring your attention back to simply sensing the area where your heart is. Reminding yourself that there is nothing in particular that you are supposed to feel when you do this practice. Just allowing your experience to be your experience.

Now you might imagine that this person or being is sending the same well-wishes to you. *May you be safe and protected. May you be happy. May you be peaceful. May you live with ease.* Noticing how that feels.

If it feels comfortable, you may shift your attention now from this being to yourself, and to sending yourself the well-wishes—*May I be safe and protected. May I be happy. May I be peaceful. May I live with ease*—or whatever wishes you have chosen, maybe just *I wish myself well—May I be happy.*

If it is easier, you may imagine yourself as a young child receiving these well-wishes. If you find yourself having judging thoughts or thinking *about* the exercise, just noticing these thoughts and guiding your attention back to the phrases. If you notice any resistance or anxiety, as best you can, allowing that resistance to soften. Seeing if you can have compassion for your experience, just as it is. Continuing to experiment with this on your own for a few more minutes.

Now, if you'd like, you might send these wishes to the people in the room with you. *May we all be safe and protected. May we be happy. May we be peaceful. May we live with ease.* Again, using whatever wishes feel most comfortable and meaningful to you. There is no need to force any particular feeling here—just simply extending wishes to yourself and the others here with you.

Take a moment to receive these wishes that the others in the room have sent to you.

Whenever you are ready, you may allow your eyes to open.

Daily Activities Worksheet
HANDOUT 7.1

A. List activities, people, and situations that you associate with **distress, challenging emotions,** or **self-doubt,** and describe how you tend to feel when you engage in these activities.

Activity, person, place, or situation	How do you tend to feel?
_____	_____
_____	_____
_____	_____
_____	_____

B. List activities, people, and situations (that don't involve substance use) that you associate with **pleasure or joy** or that increase your **confidence.** Note how you tend to feel when engaged in these activities.

Activity, person, place, or situation	How do you tend to feel?
_____	_____
_____	_____
_____	_____

Reminder Card
HANDOUT 7.2

Side One	Side Two

REASONS TO STAY ON TRACK	SOBER SPACE
•	• **S**top: pause wherever you are
•	• **O**bserve: notice what's going on right now
•	• **B**reath: direct focus to your breathing
•	• **E**xpand your awareness
•	• **R**espond with awareness

ALTERNATE ACTIVITIES/PLANS	RESOURCES
•	•
•	•
•	•
•	•
•	•

Supporting and Sustaining Well-Being
HANDOUT 7.3

THEME

We have spent several weeks bringing awareness to the specific situations, thoughts, and emotions that put us at risk for relapse. Taking care of ourselves and engaging in nourishing activities are also crucial parts of sustaining recovery. In this session, we take a look at the broader picture of our lives and identify aspects that support a healthier, more vital life as well as those that put us at risk. Lifestyle balance and compassion for oneself are essential elements of a healthy and fulfilling life.

INTEGRATING PRACTICE INTO YOUR WEEK

1. Among all the different forms of practice we have learned over the past several weeks, choose a pattern you are interested in using on a regular basis (e.g., sitting three times per week and body scan three times per week, or simply sitting six times per week). Engage in your chosen program this week.

2. Practice the SOBER space daily (regular times and whenever you notice challenging thoughts, feelings, or cravings).

3. Engage in at least three nourishing activities that you have marked on your Daily Activities Worksheet.

4. Finish filling out the reminder card, if you haven't already done so.

Daily Practice Tracking Sheet

HANDOUT 7.4

Instructions: Each day, record your mindfulness practice, also noting any barriers, observations, or comments.

Day/date	Formal practice with audio recording: How long?	SOBER space	Notes/comments
	____ minutes	How often? In what situations?	
	____ minutes	How often? In what situations?	
	____ minutes	How often? In what situations?	
	____ minutes	How often? In what situations?	
	____ minutes	How often? In what situations?	
	____ minutes	How often? In what situations?	
	____ minutes	How often? In what situations?	

SESSION 8

Social Support and Continuing Practice

This road demands courage and stamina, yet it's full of footprints.

Who are these companions?

They are rungs in your ladder. Use them!

With company you quicken your ascent.

You'll be happy enough going along, but with others, you'll get farther, and faster.

—RUMI

Materials

- Bell
- Whiteboard/markers
- Pebbles
- Handout 8.1: Resource List
- Handout 8.2: Reflections on the Course Worksheet
- Handout 8.3: Session 8 Theme: Social Support and Continuing Practice

Theme

Recovery and mindfulness practice are both lifelong journeys that require commitment and diligence. This is not an easy voyage. In fact, it can feel at times like swimming upstream. Thus far, we have learned about factors that put us at risk, some skills to help navigate through high-risk situations, and the importance of maintaining lifestyle balance. Hopefully participating in this group has also provided a sense of support and community. Having a support network is crucial to continuing along the path of practice and recovery. Recovery communities can help us recognize signs of relapse and provide support when we feel we are at risk. Having support around our meditation practice can help us sustain our practice and choose to show up for our lives in a mindful, intentional, and compassionate way.

Goals

- Highlight the importance of support networks as a way of reducing risk and maintaining recovery.

- Find ways to overcome barriers to asking for help.

- Reflect on what participants have learned from the course and reasons for continuing practice.

- Develop a plan for continued practice and incorporation of mindfulness in daily life.

Session Outline

- Check-In

- Body Scan (Practice 8.1)

- Practice Review

- The Importance of Support Networks

- Reflections on the Course

- Intentions for the Future

- Concluding Meditation (Practice 8.2)

- Closing Circle

CHECK-IN

Participants are invited to share one or two words describing a sensation, quality of mind, or emotion they are noticing. Rather than planning what they are going to say, facilitators might encourage them to listen and be present for the other group members as they share their experiences.

BODY SCAN

The body scan was practiced in the very first MBRP session. It can be useful to revisit this, giving participants a marker by which to assess changes that might have occurred over the past 2 months. Facilitators might ask about the experience of the practice and what has changed and what has stayed the same since the beginning of the course.

PRACTICE REVIEW

Practice review includes the previous week's meditation practice and a check-in on the process of establishing an individualized sustainable practice. We also review experiences with the SOBER space and with completion and use of the Reminder Card (Handout 7.2), and discuss the nourishing activities that participants chose for their home practice exercise (as described in Handout 7.3 in the section Integrating Practice into Your Week). The facilitator might ask about what participants noticed when doing these activities, the quality of their experience when engaging in the nourishing activities, and how we can bring some of those qualities into activities that feel more depleting; it is useful to reflect on how mindfulness practice can change the quality of activities and one's relationship to them. As important as reviewing participants' experiences of engaging in these activities is helping them identify barriers to engaging in nourishing activities.

THE IMPORTANCE OF SUPPORT NETWORKS

Several previous sessions explored strategies, practices, and skills for coping with stressful or risky situations. The focus then widened to include broader lifestyle choices and how those may be contributing to or detracting from our intended direction. Here we expand the lens further to look at our communities and environments (Handout 8.3).

Asking participants why support is important may seem an obvious question. It may help them to recognize, however, the crucial role of a system of support both in recovery and in sustaining a regular mindfulness practice. Neither of these paths is meant to be traveled alone; we need companions. We need encouragement and reminders to continue on this challenging journey. We often have participants offer ideas and experiences of ways to find and maintain support for both recovery and mindfulness practice. Identifying possible barriers ahead of time can be useful in recognizing and working with them if and when they arise, so we often ask participants to anticipate what might get in the way of asking for help or maintaining a support network. We also typically review current resources, such as family, friends, and 12-step or other support groups.

Finally, we offer a list of meditation resources (Handout 8.1), which can include not only websites, books, and audio resources, but also local meetings, courses, and retreats. If feasible, ongoing meditation practice sessions can be offered as part of the MBRP program, providing a safe and familiar venue to support participants' ongoing practice.

REFLECTIONS ON THE COURSE

In this final session of the course, we give participants an opportunity to reflect, individually and as a group, on their experiences over the past 2 months. We also invite them to look ahead and create an intention for continued practice. The Reflections on the Course Worksheet (Handout 8.2) asks about experiences in the course and gives participants an opportunity to provide feedback or suggestions for changes to its content and structure. We typically allow about 10 minutes for worksheet completion and remind the group that their feedback is highly valued, will remain anonymous, and will be used for the improvement of future courses.

Before collecting these sheets, we invite participants to share anything they wrote or any other reflections they might have on the course. Participants typically welcome and appreciate this opportunity to share any final thoughts, comments, or questions with the group.

INTENTIONS FOR THE FUTURE

Allowing participants to identify the importance of continued practice can be far more powerful (and interesting) than having facilitators preach the merits of daily meditation. We begin this discussion by asking the participants why they might maintain this practice, writing their ideas on the whiteboard. We often follow this by asking them to state individually what type of practice they intend to carry forward and how likely they are to continue with practice.

FACILITATOR: It will be up to each of you to decide if and how you integrate and continue mindfulness practice in your lives. If you do continue, what are some ways the practice might be helpful or important in your life?

PARTICIPANT 1: I used to make things more rigid or complicated than they needed to be, and I still do, but I can catch myself on occasion—my mind going there. This helps me stay in the here and now and not future trip or obsess about the past and get so stuck there.

PARTICIPANT 2: Keeping my awareness and being alert. Keeping my observation sharp and focused. That can tend to get dull if I don't practice. If I don't work at it, and just allow myself to be unaware, that can lead me back to relapse.

Similar to recognizing risks for relapse and identifying unhelpful patterns before they occur, it can be useful to identify barriers to continuing practice and the beginning signs of "falling off the meditation wagon":

FACILITATOR: Practice often evolves over time, so it is important to commit to practicing, and also to be aware that this is a lifetime pursuit and will go through many changes. What do you anticipate might get in the way?

PARTICIPANT 3: Time.

FACILITATOR: So finding time, setting time aside. That's a big one for people. What else?

PARTICIPANT 4: Laziness.

FACILITATOR: Okay. So what is laziness, really? What is that like or how might that play out?

PARTICIPANT 2: Like before I relapse, I stop going to meetings. I stop associating with clean people. I start doing old behaviors.

FACILITATOR: Disconnecting from the newer behaviors and falling back into old behavior patterns that are pretty familiar.

PARTICIPANT 2: Yeah. I slack off on things that I know are good or healthy for me.

FACILITATOR: So what do we do when you recognize that this is beginning to happen? We might make excuses, and maybe miss a day or two, then have that experience of the abstinence violation effect, like "I knew I couldn't do this." It's important to recognize the possibility—the probability—of this up front and to remember that we can always begin again, any day, in any moment. So if you begin to feel stuck or lose interest or find that your practice is starting to fade, what are some strategies that might help?

PARTICIPANT 2: Set a time, really schedule it into the day.

FACILITATOR: Yes. What else? What about when those excuses or that doubt comes up?

PARTICIPANT 3: Agreeing with myself that no matter what I think or how I feel, I just sit. Doing it first thing in the morning, so I just get up and sit right away without thinking too much about it.

FACILITATOR: So, making it easy for yourself. Keeping the cushion out, and audio files readily accessible, so they're right there and available. Or committing to getting into a sitting position, even if it's just for 2 minutes, just staying in the habit.

PARTICIPANT 1: Yeah, otherwise I get hard on myself, and it feels too big—"Oh, I can't this."

FACILITATOR: So even if this does happen, say a month passes and it feels way too far away, you can always begin again. You haven't "lost" it. There's no need to waste your time judging yourself. Just start again at the beginning. Always, always remembering that this practice is about compassion and about being kind to yourself. This is not another thing to beat yourself up over. This is a way to really take care of yourself, unconditionally and with a very whole and gentle compassion.

CONCLUDING MEDITATION

The concluding meditation (Practice 8.2) is intended to honor each person's journey over the past 2 months and offer a brief kindness meditation for self, fellow participants, friends and family, and finally all beings everywhere. We invite each person to choose a small stone from a collection we bring to the final group as a symbol of the rough, natural, flawed, yet perfect beauty of each human being. It is a reminder of this journey that participants can take with them to carry in a pocket or place on a desk, bedside table, or mantel.

CLOSING CIRCLE

We close the final session of the course by sitting in a circle, opening up the last moments for any final thoughts or reflections. Participants are welcome to share any final comments but are also welcome to just sit quietly. As with each of the prior sessions, the final moments are spent in silence, and the session closes with the sound of the bell.

The body scan practice from Session 1 is repeated.

Now very slowly and gently, while still maintaining an awareness of your body, when you are ready, open your eyes and allow your awareness to include the room and the rest of the people here.

Concluding Meditation
PRACTICE 8.2

Intentions

+ Recognizing that we, and others around us, are shaped by our past experiences and are a perfect part of nature just as we are
+ Practicing kindness toward self and others

I am going to come around with a bowl of stones. Please pick whatever one you are drawn to or that speaks to you.

Now as best you can, bringing all of your attention to this object, just as you did on the very first day of this course with the raisin, hold it in the palm of your hand. Examining it as though you had never seen anything like it before.

Taking a moment to turn it over, observing its color and texture, noticing places where the light hits it, noticing the sensation of it in your hand. If any thoughts come to you while you are doing this, noting and bringing your attention back to the object.

Perhaps reflect on the richness of the history—the hundreds or even thousands of years, the weather, the force of gravity—that formed this object. It has likely been subject to intense pressure from the weight above it, or tossed around in rivers or oceans. It may have been trampled on, kicked, or tossed aside. It may have also experienced times of quiet, sunlight, and stillness. All of these things have shaped it into what it is today. Noticing, too, that it isn't perfectly round, that it may have cracks and crevices, dirt or scratches on its surface. Yet it is a perfect piece of nature, just as it is.

Now holding this stone in your hand, maybe closing your hand around it, and if you'd like, allowing your eyes to gently close.

Feeling this object in your hand, and allowing it to be a reminder for you of all the things that have shaped you into who are today. You, too, have a rich history that has affected you. You, like this piece of nature in your hand, may also not be perfectly shaped. Maybe you have your own cracks and crevices, areas that have been impacted by the circumstances in your life. Yet you, like this stone, are also a perfect piece of nature. Nature is perfect in its imperfection.

Let this object be a reminder of your journey, everything that has brought you to this point in your recovery, and of continuing the process that you have started, discovering a way of being present and living alongside all the aspects of yourself, including those that may seem damaged or imperfect. Responding to them and holding them with gentleness and caring attention.

Taking a moment now to wish yourself well. If you'd like, you may focus on the well-wishes that we practiced with in the previous session and repeat them to yourself quietly, holding the stone in your hand—*May I be safe. May I be happy. May I be peaceful. May I live with ease. May I be free*—or on any other wishes that feel genuine and natural for you. What do you most wish for yourself?

Continuing to repeat these wishes a few times silently to yourself. If you find your mind wandering or notice other thoughts coming up, noting them, without judgment, and guiding your attention back to the well-wishes.

And then taking a moment to think of the person sitting to the right of you, of everything that has brought them to this point in their lives, of the struggles that they may

(continued)

have experienced along the way, and of how, like you, they are working hard to continue along this path and maintain their recovery. They, too, have had times in their life when they have been bathed in light and joy, and other times when they been enshrouded in darkness and perhaps hopelessness. They have been loved and hurt, they have felt pride and also shame. They have had times, like you, when their efforts have felt successful, and other times when they have felt defeated. So taking a moment to wish them well on their journey and offer them your wishes. *May you be safe. May you be happy. May you be peaceful. May you live with ease. May you be free.* Or whatever wishes you would like to send their way. And thinking of the person to the left of you and wishing them well. What do you wish for this person?

Now, if you'd like, expanding your awareness to include everyone in the room, and extending wishes to the whole group, including yourself. Whatever wishes you would like to silently offer. *May we all be safe, happy, peaceful, free . . .*

Now taking a moment to receive the wishes sent to you from the others here in the group, knowing that everyone here has wished you well.

Now, if you choose, expanding further to others who are important to you. Your family, your close friends, your pets. The ones you rely on, fight with, love, praise, scold, the ones you need, the ones you help. What do you wish for them? Offering them some well-wishes. *I wish you well. May you be free from suffering. May you be healthy and safe.* Whatever wishes you'd like to offer.

And finally, when you're ready, shifting awareness back to your body sitting here. Feeling the contact with the chair or cushion. The movement of breath falling in and out of the body. Feeling the stone here on your hand. Sitting quietly for a few moments, with whatever your experience is.

When you are ready—taking your time, allowing your eyes to open, and letting in the world around you.

Sections based on Segal, Williams, and Teasdale (2013).

Resource List
HANDOUT 8.1

WEBSITES

- Downloadable meditation teachings and instruction from Dharma Seed: *www.dharmaseed. org*
- Resources, meetings, podcasts, meditations: *www.refugerecovery.org*
- Local meetings and resources relevant to meditation and recovery: *www.buddhistrecovery.org*
- Guided practices, resources, clinician lists*: www.mindfulrp.com*
- Guided practices and talks: *www.tarabrach.com*

BOOKS

- *Eight Step Recovery: Using The Buddha's Teachings to Overcome Addiction, by Valerie Mason-John. Cambridge, England: Windhorse Publications, 2018.*
- *Insight Meditation: The Practice of Freedom,* by Joseph Goldstein. Boston: Shambhala, 1993.
- *The Mindful Path to Self-Compassion: Freeing Yourself from Destructive Thoughts and Emotions,* by Christopher K. Germer. New York: Guilford Press, 2009.
- *The Mindful Way through Anxiety: Break Free from Chronic Worry and Reclaim Your Life,* by Susan M. Orsillo and Lizabeth Roemer. New York: Guilford Press, 2011.
- *The Mindful Way through Depression: Freeing Yourself from Chronic Unhappiness,* by J. Mark G. Williams, John D. Teasdale, Zindel V. Segal, and Jon Kabat-Zinn. New York: Guilford Press, 2007.
- *The Miracle of Mindfulness: An Introduction to the Practice of Meditation,* by Thich Nhat Hanh. Boston: Beacon Press, 1987.
- *One Breath at a Time: Buddhism and the Twelve Steps,* by Kevin Griffin. Emmaus, PA: Rodale, 2004.
- *A Path with Heart: A Guide through the Perils and Promises of Spiritual Life,* by Jack Kornfield. New York: Bantam, 1993.
- *The Power of Meditation: A 28-Day Program, by Sharon Salzberg. New York: Workman Publishing, 2010.*
- *Radical Acceptance: Embracing Your Life with the Heart of a Buddha,* by Tara Brach. New York: Bantam, 2003.
- *Seeking the Heart of Wisdom: The Path of Insight Meditation,* by Joseph Goldstein and Jack Kornfield. Boston: Shambhala, 1987.
- *Start Where You Are: A Guide to Compassionate Living,* by Pema Chödrön. Boston: Shambhala, 1994.
- *10% Happier: How I Tamed the Voice in My Head, Reduced Stress without Losing My Edge, and Found Self-Help That Actually Works,* by Dan Harris. New York: Dey Street, 2014.
- *True Refuge: Finding Peace and Freedom in Your Own Awakened Heart, by Tara Brach. New York: Bantam, 2013.*
- *When Things Fall Apart: Heart Advice for Difficult Times,* by Pema Chödrön. Boston: Shambhala, 1997.
- *Wherever You Go, There You Are: Mindfulness Meditation in Everyday Life,* by Jon Kabat-Zinn. New York: Hyperion, 1994.

Please take a moment to reflect upon the following questions and write down your responses:

1. What did you find most valuable about this course? What, if anything, did you learn?

2. What, if anything, has changed for you during the course as a result of your participation?

3. Was there anything that got in the way of your learning or growth or that might have improved the course for you?

4. Other comments?

5. On a scale of 1 (*not at all*) to 10 (*very*), how important has this program been to you? Please explain why you have given it this rating.

6. On a scale of 1 (*not at all*) to 10 (*very*), how likely are you to continue engaging in **formal** mindfulness practice (e.g., body scan, sitting meditation, mindful stretching/movement) after this course?

7. On a scale of 1 (*not at all*) to 10 (*very*), how likely are you to continue engaging in **informal** mindfulness practice (e.g., SOBER space, mindful eating, walking, daily activities) after this course?

Session 8 Theme
Social Support and Continuing Practice
HANDOUT 8.3

Using the mindfulness skills we've learned in this course can help us face our experiences differently; we can accept the experience instead of fighting it, and from there make choices from a wiser, more spacious place. This moment-by-moment journey of recovery and mindfulness practice can feel, at times, like swimming upstream. It is not an easy voyage. But we are fully capable of it.

Thus far, we have learned about the factors that put us at risk, some skills to help navigate through high-risk situations, and the importance of maintaining overall well-being. Participating in this group has also hopefully offered a sense of support and community. Having a support network is crucial to continuing along the path of practice and recovery. It can help us recognize signs of relapse and provide encouragement when we feel we are at risk. Having support around our meditation practice can help us maintain our practice and choose to show up for our lives.

There are many things we do not have control over and many things that may not go "our way." We do have a choice, however, in how we respond and how we experience our lives. Practicing mindfulness on a regular basis helps us be less reactive and more aware in our choices, ultimately giving us greater freedom. Taking care of ourselves and engaging in activities that nourish us is part of maintaining balance in our lives and helping protect against relapse. Maintaining a practice is not easy. Difficulties and barriers will arise. Be gentle with yourself. Remember that any practice is good practice; you can always begin again from right where you are.

PART III

Research and Adaptations

Twenty years ago, research on mindfulness and addictions was virtually nonexistent. Today, studies assessing efficacy, underlying mechanisms, and adaptations of mindfulness-based approaches for treating addictive behaviors number in the hundreds, reflecting interest in and commitment to new approaches in addiction treatment, and recognition that ancient wisdom and current science can indeed inform and support one another.

These studies fall into five basic categories: (1) cross-sectional designs, assessing relationships between trait levels of mindfulness and craving or addictive behaviors; (2) studies assessing feasibility and efficacy of mindfulness training for treatment of addictive behaviors; (3) mechanisms underlying changes that occur in mindfulness-based interventions (i.e., how or why mindfulness training affects addictive behavior); (4) factors that influence treatment effects such as gender or addiction severity; and (5) adaptations or revisions to intervention protocols to better suit specific contexts or cultures. These categories reflect the progression common in clinical research and are clearly represented in research relevant to this approach. One body of studies assessed relationships between mindfulness traits or processes and addictive behavior. In light of evidence indicating that higher levels of mindful awareness and/or mindful action are related to decreased risk or severity of substance use, another body of studies assessed how to foster mindfulness traits, practices, or views to help reduce addictive behaviors. Given the promise of these studies, interest then included mechanisms, or active change ingredients, to better understand the processes underlying these changes in primary outcomes. Finally, now that significant evidence supports these approaches and we are beginning to understand why or how change occurs, more recent studies are assessing their appropriateness and availability across diverse contexts and populations. This includes assessment of who is benefiting, and who perhaps isn't,

171

to inform future adaptations or revisions to practices, language or other intervention characteristics to better suit a broader population.

While numerous studies support the first stage of this research, suggesting an inverse relationship between levels of mindfulness and addictive behaviors and/or their correlates, the following sections focus on the latter four categories of study, namely feasibility and effects of mindfulness training on substance use-related outcomes, understanding the mechanisms of change underlying these effects, assessing for whom treatment is effective, and adaptations to better suit a broader diversity of population.

EARLY RESEARCH ON THE EFFICACY OF MEDITATION FOR TREATMENT OF ADDICTIVE BEHAVIOR

The earliest studies of meditation and addictive behaviors were primarily focused on Transcendental Meditation (TM), a tradition created in the mid-1950s that differed from mindfulness meditation primarily in its focus on a word or sound, called a mantra, repeated by the meditator to support concentration. The first trials in this sequence were with college student drinkers, and showed consistent reductions in alcohol use following a mantra-based meditation similar to TM, with an average 50% decrease in daily drinking (Marlatt et al., 1984), and evidence suggesting both meditation and physical exercise were helpful in reducing alcohol consumption in male college students (Murphy, Pagano, & Marlatt, 1986). Alongside these early trials, over 30 studies investigated the effectiveness of TM in the treatment of substance use disorder. Overall, these studies demonstrated positive effects of TM in reducing alcohol and drug use (see Alexander, Robinson, Orme-Johnson, & Schneider, 1994, for a review). Results from these studies supported feasibility and acceptance of meditation as an intervention and suggested that it may be effective for college students and other "heavy social drinkers." This was the beginning of what would become a long series of clinical trials assessing meditation practices for treatment of addictive behaviors.

Though the roots and practices of TM differ from those of mindfulness practices, this early research laid the groundwork for integrating meditation practices into cognitive-behavioral treatment for addictive behaviors. The foundations of the meditation practices in MBRP come from the ancient practice of vipassana. Although vipassana dates back thousands of years, traditional Western psychology and medicine have only recently begun to integrate similar practices into treatment protocols. As in MBRP, contemporary implementations of practices are typically in secular form to better suit modern-day medical contexts.

A seminal article published in the beginning stages of the vipassana and mindfulness-based research (Marlatt, 2002) describes addiction as stemming from a mistaken understanding of substance use as a true refuge from suffering, in contrast to conceptualizing or treating addiction as a moral shortcoming, as it had often been viewed in the past. The article described how mindfulness practice can address the roots of craving and reactive behaviors, and the parallels between meditation practice and CBT (cognitive-behavioral therapy). Mindfulness practice allows the practitioner to directly observe the mind's behavior, and to self-monitor thoughts and feelings with acceptance and nonjudgmental objectivity. Marlatt considered these practices "essential to understanding how the mind behaves and how thoughts and expectations can either facilitate or reduce the occurrence of addictive behavior" (Marlatt, 2002, p. 49).

The first major trial assessing the effects of vipassana meditation on addictive behaviors came in the late 1990s to early 2000s. A study of adult residents at a minimum-security jail who were participating in an intensive 10-day vipassana course, taught in its traditional Buddhist form, showed evidence of significant improvements in substance use as well as positive psychosocial outcomes when compared with participants in the treatment-as-usual condition (Bowen et al., 2006). Specifically, 3 months following release from jail, those who had taken the course, compared to inmates who did not, reported significantly less alcohol and drug use and significantly fewer related negative consequences.

Recognizing barriers to participation in an intensive residential 10-day Buddhist meditation retreat, Marlatt and several students in his lab began to design a secularized program more feasible for community settings, and one in which the practice of observing one's experience—including thoughts, emotions, sensations, and behaviors—wasn't affiliated with any religion or even tradition. This method of directly observing and developing insight into one's experiences and behavior patterns can be taught in a way that is accessible to people of all backgrounds, religions, contexts, cultures, and levels of education. Marlatt's team constructed a program using a framework similar to those of the pioneering MBSR and MBCT programs, two recently developed evidence-based treatment approaches integrating mindfulness meditation into treatment approaches. This work resulted in the 8-week outpatient aftercare program mindfulness-based relapse prevention (MBRP).

RESEARCH ON MBRP

Feasibility, Efficacy, and Mechanisms Underlying Change

The initial randomized controlled trial of MBRP was conducted in a community-based treatment agency in an urban setting. Study participants ($N = 168$) had completed inpatient or intensive outpatient treatment and were transitioning into an aftercare phase. Participants reported a range of primary substances of abuse, the most common of which was alcohol (45%), followed by cocaine/crack (36%), methamphetamines (14%), opiates/heroin (7%), marijuana (5%), and other (2%). Approximately 19% were polysubstance users. Participants were randomized to either the 8-week MBRP program or to continuation of treatment as usual (TAU), which consisted of 12-step approaches, process groups, and psychoeducation.

At a 2-month follow-up assessment, participants in MBRP reported significantly greater decreases in substance use compared to those in TAU. They also reported greater reductions in craving, which in turn partially mediated (or explained) the reductions in substance use. Additionally, MBRP participants reported greater increases in awareness and acceptance (Bowen et al., 2009) and showed a decrease in the strength of the relation between depressive symptoms and subsequent craving compared to TAU participants (Witkiewitz & Bowen, 2010). This suggested that they were less likely to experience a craving response in reaction to negative affective states, one of the primary precipitants of relapse (Marlatt & Donovan, 2005).

The next major trial, several years later, again compared MBRP and TAU but added a cognitive-behavioral relapse prevention (RP) comparison condition. The trial also included a larger number of participants and extended the follow-up window to 12 months following end of treatment to better assess relative sustainability of treatment gains. Results showed that participants in both MBRP and RP, as compared to TAU, had significantly lower risk of relapse to substance use and heavy drinking and, among those who used substances, significantly fewer days of substance use and heavy drinking at a 6-month follow-up. At the 12-month follow-up, however, only MBRP (vs. both RP and TAU) showed lower likelihood of relapse and significantly fewer days of substance use or heavy drinking (Bowen et al., 2014). Follow-up studies have identified mechanisms underlying changes seen in these trials, such as maladaptive responses to negative affect and craving (Witkiewitz & Bowen, 2010; Enkema & Bowen, 2017; Witkiewitz, Bowen, Douglas, & Hsu, 2013).

Differential Treatment Effects
and the Need for Cultural and Contextual Adaptations

Taking a broad view of the past 20 years of work in this field, we are now at a point at which focus is shifting from studying efficacy of this approach to understanding and maximizing the effects of MBRP. Advancements in our own work and in the broader field move us toward more sensitive and effective adaptations for other cultures and individuals with marginalized backgrounds, distinct contexts, and more complex individual psychological profiles. Thus, a newer line of research is assessing differential effects of treatment by factors such as race/ethnicity and gender (Greenfield et al., 2018; Witkiewitz, Greenfield, & Bowen, 2013) and comorbid affective disorders (Glasner et al., 2017; Roos, Bowen, & Witkiewitz, in press; Witkiewitz & Bowen, 2010).

Other recent trials are assessing feasibility and efficacy of revisions to the initial protocol format to better suit the structures and strictures of the settings in which they are implemented. Two recent studies assessed a rolling admission format, instead of the original closed-cohort structure, to allow patients at these clinics to enter the treatment groups at any time. In one such study, women in a residential criminal justice addictions treatment program were randomized to 8 weeks of a rolling admission MBRP group and compared to participants in standard RP. Those in the MBRP group reported significantly fewer days of drug use and fewer legal and medical problems at a 15-week follow-up (Witkiewitz et al., 2014). Another recent trial assessed a twice-weekly rolling admission format (Roos et al., 2018), with results supporting feasibility, acceptability and efficacy of this format.

The structure of the program has also been modified to better serve specific patient populations, including those with behavioral addictions such as gambling and eating disorders, the deaf population, first responders, and, in perhaps the fastest-growing body of work, individuals with co-occurring PTSD and substance use disorder. Recent trials have also explored adaptations for international populations (Curado et al., 2018) and implementation in prison settings (Lyons, Womack, Cantrell, & Kenemore, 2019) and with young adults in residential treatment (Davis et al., 2019). Across all of the diverse populations, what remains central is the intention of the practices and the program—to help participants better see for themselves the internal processes that underlie and perpetuate problematic behaviors. Below we describe issues to consider when adapting and implementing the program in cultures and settings other than the ones in which it was originally created.

Considerations When Adapting the Program

While we understand and appreciate the value of a standard protocol as a way to share and assess this approach, we also recognize that the context in which the program was originally formed may differ from other contexts, settings, and cultures with their unique needs.

This program, like those after which it was modeled, was developed within a Western psychological, scientific, and cultural framework. The program represents the developers' interpretation of ancient practices through this lens and world view. While the practices themselves have a certain timelessness and simplicity, it is important to acknowledge that this program may require adaptations and modifications depending on the culture and context in which it is being implemented. Rather than assuming the program described in these pages is immutable, we have encouraged facilitators and those who may be adapting it to be flexible with the form of the program, paying attention to the needs of their participants while adhering to the underlying intention of each exercise. As with any intervention, it is helpful for facilitators to either be part of the community with whom they are working with or to have an informed understanding of the nuances and dynamics of the culture.

MBRP was created and initially implemented in the United States. However, over the past decade, the program has been adapted for and implemented in numerous other countries, and the protocol has been translated into several different languages, including German, Chinese, Spanish, and Portuguese. Over the past decade, we have explored multiple revisions and adaptations to best fit a variety of diverse contexts. We have also learned from colleagues who further broaden the scope of these applications. Our intent has been, in our own work and with the clinicians we have trained, to keep at the center the intentions of the program. However, the form of the course, the language, and the practices are flexible, as long as they are training the processes underlying behaviors we aim to target.

Not only is it important for those who are adapting this program internationally to consider particular sociopolitical contexts, but even on a very practical level, certain wording, references, metaphors, and exercises may not have the same significance in another context or culture. One illustrative example occurred at a facilitator training workshop with a participant who hoped to adapt the program for use in another country. She brought up questions about the raisin exercise, used as an experiential introduction to mindfulness in a variety of mindfulness programs with the intention of bringing awareness to something relatively mundane that, when attention is given to it, offers significant sensory input and illustrates our tendency toward autopilot. However, in this participant's culture, a raisin was not a familiar food, and thus while the novelty of the experience may provide sensory information and invite curiosity, the practice may not serve the same intention. The facilitator substituted a different food item, while holding to the underlying intention of the practice.

A further example is use of the mountain metaphor. A group of clinicians working at a treatment agency in the southeastern United States found that many participants were unable to picture or relate to the image or qualities of a mountain, some having never seen one. In their geographical region, the ancient, towering oak trees were far more salient. They thus adapted the practice using the deep-rootedness, strong yet flexible trunk and branches, and majestic stance of an oak tree as a way to connect with these qualities in themselves.

Similar consideration may be required with other exercises such as urge surfing, given that a surfing metaphor may not be accessible or relatable for everyone. Again, the intention behind using metaphors is what is important to understand, that is, in urge surfing we are practicing staying in contact with a challenging experience and riding it through, versus fighting it or being lost in it. This can be communicated in many ways, with or without the term "surfing." Similarly, certain words, when translated into other languages, may not have the same connotation and may require modification. It may also be helpful to supplement the handouts or replace poems with material by authors and poets who are part of the cultural context.

A significant challenge to implementation is access to necessary resources. A recent study in Brazil (Opaleye, Machado, Bowen, & Noto, 2019), the first implementation study of MBRP in a Latin American country, assessed barriers to implementation across multiple community treatment sites in São Paulo. Primary barriers included access to professional clinician training, necessary changes to the MBRP course format (increasing duration of the course, decreasing length of sessions, and altering the order of some activities), and need for a "rolling group" protocol to allow patients to join at different points in the course to better suit the many logistical challenges they face in beginning and sustaining treatment.

Finally, cultural adaptations may involve connecting meditation to, or ensuring it is not in conflict with, familiar religious and spiritual practices and ideologies. Although mindfulness practices are designed to be secular, there may be participants who feel that these practices are religiously incongruent. It may be helpful for facilitators to support an open conversation about how mindfulness may conflict with the spirituality or religious beliefs of participants, and to explore ways in which mindfulness practices can enhance or complement other religious or spiritual practices.

As this program continues to expand its implementation and refine its form, we encourage and look forward to adaptations and revisions to better serve cultures and contexts other than those in which the program was originally created. In the Appendix, we offer a handout ("Intentions of MBRP Exercises and Practices") to help facilitators keep at the center of their work the function, or intention, of each of the main practices in the program, even though the form of the guidance may change to better reach or more appropriately share these practices and ideas with diverse populations to whom they should be available.

ALTERNATIVE STRUCTURES AND FORMATS

This section provides descriptions and examples of modifications to the MBRP structure and format to suit the needs of contexts that vary from the one within which the program was originally. They include the addition of an introductory session prior to the 8-week program, use of a rolling group format, an extra session for extended mindfulness practice, and a 6-week version of the program.

Introductory Session

Offering an introductory session prior to Week 1 of a course that follows the MBRP protocol can serve multiple purposes. In two studies (Bowen et al., 2009; Somohano, Manuel, Rutkie, & Bowen, 2016), participants were offered an individual brief introductory session in which they discussed motivations, concerns, and potential barriers to participating in the group. In the style and spirit of motivational interviewing (MI; Miller & Rollnick, 2013), this was intended to allow potential participants to express doubts or ambivalence about being in the group, and to support their intrinsic motivation for participation. Another study, currently under way, assessing an adapted MBRP course for women with comorbid PTSD and substance use disorder (Killeen, Feigl, Shaw, & Bowen, 2018), is implementing a 2-hour group-based introductory session prior to the beginning of the course. The session is offered by the MBRP facilitator and is conducted using a style similar to MI. Participants are asked about their experiences with PTSD symptomology, the relationship between that and their substance use patterns, and how mindfulness practices (introduced using a video) might be useful in concurrently addressing both PTSD and addiction. They have an opportunity to ask questions about the upcoming 8-week course.

Closed versus Rolling Enrollment

As currently designed, MBRP is delivered in a "closed" group format, with all participants beginning together at Session 1 and finishing together at Session 8. The practices are designed to build upon one another, and thus sessions are kept in sequence. However, as mentioned above, we and some of our colleagues have been experimenting with different formats—for example, admitting new participants at Week 4, with the addition of an introductory session exclusively for the new participants (Brewer et al., 2009), or implementing a "rolling" course design, wherein participants can enter or exit the group at any session (Roos et al., 2018). Although a closed group format, with members experiencing the full 8-week course together, offers many benefits, a rolling format may permit more clients to participate in the course and allow "experienced" participants to inform and support the newer group members. This may be essential in treatment centers with higher volumes of ongoing admissions, allowing participants to enter and/or exit the group at any time, versus only at the beginning and end of an 8-week period.

Below is a sample format for a rolling group (Roos et al., 2018):

Included in Every Session

1. Expectations and Describing the Group
2. Mindful Check-In

3. Inquiry Following Mindful Check-In

4. Discussion: What is mindfulness? How does it relate to recovery?

5. Session end: Review new practices/skills covered during session, suggest practice outside session

Individual Modules

1. Stepping Out of Autopilot
   - Raisin/mindful eating exercise and inquiry
   - Teach, practice, discuss SOBER space

2. Mindfulness and Thoughts
   - Brief thoughts exercise, what are thoughts, and thoughts meditation
   - "Walking down the street" and inquiry
   - Breath meditation and inquiry

3. Mindfulness and Valued Living
   - Mindful movement and inquiry (in place of mindful check-in)
   - Introduce SOBER space
   - Values worksheet, meditation, and inquiry

4. Why We Practice
   - Body scan and inquiry (in place of mindful check-in)
   - False refuge
   - Developing a practice, common challenges

5. Self-Compassion
   - Kindness meditation and inquiry

6. Mindfulness in Challenging Situations
   - SOBER practice discussion
   - SOBER in pairs and inquiry

7. Mindfulness and Emotions
   - Brief practice and reading of guest-house poem, then inquiry

8. Checking in during Difficult Moments
   - Discuss relationship between sensations/emotions/thoughts/actions
   - Checking in during a difficult moment (i.e., urge surfing) and inquiry

Extended Mindfulness Practice Session

Many mindfulness-based interventions include an extended session of practice intended to give participants an opportunity to deepen practice using a retreat-like structure. Although we were not able to offer this as part of the MBRP clinical trials, due to limitations on space and other logistics at the agency where the trial was conducted, we have offered a half-day (or longer) "retreat" for extended mindfulness practice in nonresearch contexts. These sessions are typically held on a weekend morning, either between Sessions 5 and 6, or Sessions 6 and 7. Alternating between periods of sitting meditation and either walking meditation or mindful movement, the session is held primarily in silence, without conversation, inquiry, or engagement with technological devices during breaks. The session often ends with kindness practice, if that has already been introduced, coming out of silence, and a period of reflection and Q&A.

It is advisable to let participants know about the structure and expectations of the half day of mindfulness in advance, including the intentions of holding silence. It is especially helpful to explain that the silence is not intended to be oppressive, but rather an opportunity to free ourselves from the burden of social expectations and as a way to respect each other's processes during this retreat time. Any reactions related to this are welcome and interesting to observe, and can be discussed at the end of the day's session. It can also help to clarify that participants are welcome to check in with the facilitator(s) at any time, especially if they are struggling with any part of their experience.

A sample 3- or 4-hour session might look like this:

- Welcome, review of silence instructions, and rationale
- Sitting practice
- Walking practice
- Silent break
- Sitting practice
- Walking practice
- Silent break
- Kindness practice
- Reflection, Q&A
- Closing practice

Six-Week Format

We have on occasion offered a modified 6- versus 8-week version of the program. While a few practices are folded together, the format maintains all of the core components of the program. Sessions are slightly longer, at 2½ hours long.

Below is an example of this format.

Session 1: Automatic Pilot and Relapse

- Introductions
- Expectations for Group/Confidentiality
- Group Structure and Format
- Raisin Exercise/Automatic Pilot and Relapse
- What Is Mindfulness?
- Body Scan
- Home Practice

Session 2: Triggers and Craving

- Check-In
- Sitting Meditation: Sound, Breath
- Home Practice Review and Common Challenges
- Walking Down the Street Exercise
- Urge Surfing and Discussion of Craving
- Mountain Meditation
- Home Practice
- Closing

Session 3: From Reacting to Responding

- Check-In
- Sitting Meditation: Sound, Breath, Sensation, Thought
- Home Practice Review
- High-Risk Situations; False Refuge Exercise
- SOBER
- SOBER in a Challenging Situation
- Walking Meditation
- Home Practice
- Closing

Session 4: Thoughts

- Check-In
- Brief Discussion of Thoughts; Sitting Meditation: Thoughts
- Home Practice Review
- Thoughts and Relapse
- Relapse Chain
- SOBER in Pairs
- Mindful Movement or Walking Meditation
- Home Practice
- Closing

Session 5: Emotion

- Check-In
- Sitting: Sound, Breath, Sensation, Thought, Emotion (with Rumi Poem)
- Practice Review
- Acceptance and Skillful Action Discussion
- Kindness Meditation
- Home Practice
- Closing

Session 6: Self-Care/ Lifestyle Balance and Continuing Practice

- Check-In
- Body Scan (with Poem)
- Practice Review
- Daily Activities Worksheet
- Importance of Support Networks/Discuss Resources
- Intentions for Future
- Reflections on Course
- Concluding Meditation/Closing

ENSURING TREATMENT INTEGRITY

Part I of this book discusses the background and training recommended for facilitators of mindfulness-based interventions, emphasizing the importance of interventionists having their own formal mindfulness practice, and describes primary intentions of the program and the components of the inquiry process. However, it is not uncommon for facilitators to drift from these principles over time, or to revert to familiar methods of group facilitation that may be inconsistent with this approach. Thus, it is helpful to have a tool to assess fidelity and, when possible, couple this with ongoing supervision. In a research context, a measure of treatment integrity can be helpful in training and supervising facilitators; ensuring the validity of treatment study findings (Bellg et al., 2004); detecting differences or shifts in adherence, or the extent to which interventions and approaches that are prescribed are delivered and those that are proscribed are avoided; and measuring competence, or the skill with which interventionists deliver the treatment (Waltz, Addis, Koerner, & Jacobson, 1993).

As part of the initial randomized controlled trial of MBRP, we developed a preliminary measure (fidelity scale) of therapist adherence and competence in delivering MBRP and used it to assess the extent to which therapists in the initial trial adhered to protocol and demonstrated competence in treatment delivery (Chawla et al., 2010). After many subsequent trials, this tool has been revised. While it continues to be a work in progress as our own understanding and experience continue to mature, the current revised version is included in the Appendix for those who wish to use it in their own training and implementation efforts. It is designed to assess core components of inquiry, as well as critical facilitation skills.

TECHNOLOGY AND AUDIOVISUAL RESOURCES

Having developed this program over a decade ago, we have seen significant changes in potentially supportive technology. For example, when the original program was created, smartphones and tablets were brand new, mobile app stores were just being developed, and web-based distribution of meditation instruction audio files was rare. Such resources can now offer supplemental support to MBRP participants as they move through the program. We encourage use of these, as long as they are serving to increase access or understanding, or support practice or engagement consistent with MBRP. For example, some facilitators post their practice recordings on a website and e-mail a link to participants, while others suggest mobile apps consistent with the style of MBRP practices. As of this writing, a number of mindfulness apps exist, many more are being developed, and all are ever changing. There are several apps that record frequency and duration of playback of the audio instructions, and these may help participants, facilitators, and researchers see patterns of practice. Finally, several facilitators have experimented with live online MBRP groups, using web-conferencing software.

Videos have also proven useful in MBRP. In Session 3, we used to show videos of other mindfulness-based courses, selecting ones relevant to the specific population we were currently serving. For example, certain groups with a history of incarceration responded well to *Changing from Inside* (Donnenfield, 1998), a documentary that follows a 10-day vipassana meditation course conducted in a Seattle, Washington, jail with individuals incarcerated for drug-related charges. We have also used "Healing from Within," an episode of the Bill Moyers series *Healing and the Mind* that includes video from one of Jon Kabat-Zinn's MBSR classes. Participants seem able to draw parallels between living with chronic pain and living with addiction and ongoing cravings and urges. The videos often bring an added appreciation and understanding of the process in the absence of seeing others who have been through the course.

In other groups, we have used more contemporary video segments, such as the recent *60 Minutes* segment about mindfulness meditation with Anderson Cooper. This has been shown as part of an introductory session prior to beginning the 8-week MBRP course. In many groups, however, we have chosen to exclude video altogether. We suggest facilitators reconsider the usefulness of this type of support. For participants who have more familiarity with, or motivation for, meditation practice, it may be less appropriate.

Intentions of MBRP Exercises and Practices

Note: Primary intentions are set in **bold** text.

SESSION 1: AUTOMATIC PILOT AND MINDFUL AWARENESS

Raisin Exercise

- **Experientially discern between "automatic pilot" and mindful awareness**
- Explore relationship between automatic/reactive behavior and substance use/relapse
- Introduce mindfulness by bringing all senses to an external, tangible object

What Is Mindfulness?

- **Allow participants to describe/define mindfulness based on direct experience with raisin exercise**
- Highlight nonjudgment as an aspect of mindful awareness

Body Scan

- **Awareness of body sensations as a way to directly connect with present-moment experience**
- Openness and curiosity toward all experiences, versus expectations about what "should" or "shouldn't" be happening
- Exploring relevance of paying attention to physical experience and reactivity, cravings, and urges
- Shifting focus of attentional training from the outside object (raisin) to an interoceptive awareness of the body, and intentionally moving awareness from one area of focus to the next

(continued)

SESSION 2: A NEW RELATIONSHIP WITH DISCOMFORT

Common Challenges

These challenges often arise and are commonly viewed as "problems," though they are universal.

- **Shifting one's relationship to these challenges, recognizing them as common experiences to acknowledge and possibly even befriend ("inviting in" the visitors, as in the Rumi poem)**

Walking Down the Street Exercise

- **Observing the tendency for proliferation of thoughts, emotions, physical sensations, and urges to react in response to the *interpretation of* an ambiguous event**
- Noticing and recognizing them as such, rather than as the "truth"
- Beginning to differentiate thoughts, emotions, physical sensations, and urges and noticing how they affect (or "feed") one another
- Noticing if reactions are familiar, and thus beginning to recognize cognitive or behavioral patterns in response to triggers

Urge Surfing

- **Exposure/response prevention: Staying present with and observe the experience of craving/urges with kindness and curiosity, without engaging in reactive or resistant behavior**
- Exploring the experience of craving, including physical sensations, thoughts, and urges, therefore dismantling an experience that often feels overwhelming and typically elicits reactivity
- Looking "beneath" the craving for underlying, often wholesome, needs (e.g., relief from difficult emotions, a desire for peace or freedom)

Mountain Meditation

- **Embodying the stabilizing, grounded, rooted, and still qualities of a mountain, even in the face of inner and outer "weather" (e.g., changing circumstances, challenging situations or emotions)**
- Knowing that we have these inner resources available to us at any time

(continued)

186

SESSION 3: FROM REACTING TO RESPONDING

Awareness of Hearing

- **Bringing awareness to sensory experience versus content**
- Noticing the mind's tendency to immediately jump in to assess, label, categorize, and judge, and how this can obstruct our true vision or raw experience
- Offering a practice that can help us "get out of our heads"

Breath Meditation

- **Practicing repeatedly returning focus to a present-centered experience (breath)**
- Noticing the tendency of the mind to wander and get caught in thoughts and stories, and practicing nonjudgmental awareness
- Disabusing ourselves of ideas about meditation being a "trancelike" state, or a relaxation exercise

False Refuge

- Recognizing needs that often underlie craving
- Exploring whether addictive behavior truly fulfills these underlying needs
- Recognizing addictive behavior as a misguided way of getting our needs met

SOBER Space

- **Integrating mindfulness into daily life by practicing the shift out of "autopilot" and into awareness, especially in situations in which we tend to be reactive**
- Establishing a clear, focused, and portable practice for higher-stress situations
- Observing whatever is arising—not necessarily changing our experience or "feeling better"—which may allow for choice in the face of challenging situations

(continued)

SESSION 4: MINDFULNESS IN CHALLENGING SITUATIONS

Awareness of Seeing

- Observing present experience through a different "sense door"

- **Noticing deeply habitual ways in which the mind works (i.e., "automatically" labeling and categorizing), and how this can obstruct our true vision or raw experience**

Sitting Meditation (Sound, Breath, Sensation, Thought)

- Expanding the field of awareness to include other sense experiences

- **Becoming aware that all sense experiences are in the same class. Rather than thoughts or emotions being more important or true, all these experiences arise and pass in our field of awareness, moment to moment**

- Practicing observation of physical and emotional discomfort, and meeting it with patience, curiosity, and kindness, rather than with resistance

- Further noticing the mind's tendency to automatically label, categorize, and judge

Individual and Common Relapse Risks

- **Awareness of individual risks and relapse patterns, and of the commonality of these factors and challenges**

- Specific focus on how mindfulness practices might be useful in high-risk situations

Sober in a Challenging Situation

- **Pausing at the brink of where we typically become reactive, and practicing presence and awareness versus reacting on autopilot**

- Learning that it is possible to "stay," even when it feels intolerable

- Exploring our experience with curiosity and kindness

- Experiencing how greater awareness of experience just as it is can allow the space necessary to make a more mindful, intentional choice

Walking Meditation

- **Bringing attention to the body in motion, grounding oneself in physical sensations**

- Increasing awareness of another often "automatic" daily activity

- Noticing the experience of just walking versus trying to get somewhere (i.e., being vs. doing)

(continued)

SESSION 5: ACCEPTANCE AND SKILLFUL ACTION

Sitting Meditation (Sound, Breath, Sensation, Thought, Emotion)

- Experiencing emotion as another arising (and passing) event—with sensory and cognitive elements

- **Noticing raw elements of emotion versus stories about it or reactivity to it**

Sober Space in Pairs

- **Generalizing SOBER practice to everyday challenges by inducing a slightly more agitated, distracted, or "automatic" mode**

- Practicing mindful pausing in the context of an interpersonal exchange

Discussion of Acceptance and Skillful Action

- **Accepting what already *is* versus wishing things were different (fighting against reality)**

- Accepting things as they are—providing a stable, clear vision from which to make change in the future

Mindful Movement

- **Another modality of mindfulness practice: repeatedly returning attention to sensations in the body while in motion and engaging in different postures, distinguished from trying to "achieve" something**

- Noticing emotional responses in relation to the body (e.g., urges to escape discomfort, self-judgment, and evaluation)

- Befriending the body by making space for emotional and physical discomfort, as well as pleasant sensations and a sense of well-being (listening to the body, respecting what it says)

(continued)

SESSION 6: SEEING THOUGHTS AS THOUGHTS

Sitting Meditation: Thoughts

- **Observing thoughts similarly to how we have been observing sounds and sensation—arising and passing objects of attention**

- Creating distance and perspective by observing thoughts as objects, while stepping back from their content, using metaphors to observe the arising and passing of thoughts in the mind

- Thoughts as simply words or images arising in the mind, rather than reliable reflections of "truth"

- Recognizing judgment as yet another thought

Relapse Cycle

- **Disaggregating the seemingly automatic process of relapse**

- **Realizing that slowing down and observing thoughts, emotions, and sensations can allow us to step out of the "automatic" cycle and choose a more skillful response**

- Decentering from thoughts that may lead to relapse through recognition and familiarity

- Distinguishing a lapse from the full-blown cycle of relapse and illustrating the many points of choice following a lapse

- Discussing the abstinence violation effect, and exploring individual "relapse signatures" as a way to prepare and minimize damage

(continued)

SESSION 7: SUPPORTING AND SUSTAINING WELL-BEING

Kindness Meditation

- **Practicing kindness toward self and others**
- **Observing whatever arises** in the practice (including resistance and aversion) with openness and curiosity, rather than expecting a particular feeling or sentiment

Daily Activities Worksheet

- Bringing awareness to ordinary daily activities and how they tend to affect overall mood, life balance, and health
- Recognizing not just the categories of things that tend to be nourishing or depleting, but also the qualities (e.g., "I feel depleted when I'm pressured and I feel nourished when I have a sense of freedom," compared with "I feel depleted at work")
- Noticing balance between depleting versus nourishing activities, and the importance of including nourishing activities
- **How we relate to "depleting" activities can make them more or less depleting**
- **Not missing the pleasurable experiences in our lives—being present for the nourishing activities**
- Recognizing how ways we relate to daily activities, and the imbalance between nourishment/depletion, can put us at higher risk for relapse

(continued)

191

SESSION 8: SOCIAL SUPPORT AND CONTINUING PRACTICE

Importance of Support

- Recognizing the importance of a support network, for maintaining both mindfulness practice and recovery

- **Identifying excuses/barriers to seeking support and discussing possible actions to overcome these**

Reflections on the Course

- **Recognizing which aspects/practices have been beneficial and ways this practice has supported recovery and greater life goals/values**

- Opportunity to share experience and provide feedback

Intentions for the Future

- **Articulating plans for integrating practice into daily life (e.g., types of practices, time of day)**

Closing Circle/Concluding Meditation

- Recognizing that we, and others around us, are shaped by our past experiences and are a perfect part of nature just as we are

- Practicing kindness toward self and others

Mindfulness-Based Relapse Prevention—Fidelity Scale

A. INQUIRY				
Facilitating inquiry and responding to questions or comments	Absent	Minimal	Adequate	Superior
1. **Awareness of Current Experience:** What did you notice? Encourages awareness of present moment experience. Elicits/highlights experiences. (*"What did you notice?" "Did you notice anything in your body?" "So you noticed the thought that . . . " "Anyone notice the mind wandering?"*)	0	1	2	3
2. **Curiosity:** Exploring the experience Encourages further exploration, curiosity, and nonjudgment toward what is noticed. (*"What is the experience of anger like for you? Where do you feel it?" "What does an itch really feel like? Is it burning, hot, pulsing, throbbing?"*)	0	1	2	3
3. **Acceptance:** How are you relating to the experience? What was it like to be with that? Highlights or inquires about the difference between relating to experiences with acceptance versus aversion or grasping. (*Allowing and being with difficult emotional and physical states versus trying to get rid of them or manipulate one's experience in some way*)	0	1	2	3
4. **Familiar or Different** Inquires about whether an experience is familiar (i.e., habitual/autopilot) or different (i.e., raw experience, mindful awareness).	0	1	2	3
5. **Relevance/Relation** Explores how practices or in-session experiences relate to behavior, daily life, or addiction.	0	1	2	3

(continued)

B. GUIDING PRACTICE

	Unsatisfactory		Satisfactory		Excellent
Adapting to present context Pacing, inclusion/adaptation of instructions as needed (*Ambient noise, participant experiences, challenges with practice, etc.*)	0	1	2	3	4

C. GENERAL SKILLS

		Unsatisfactory		Satisfactory		Excellent
Attitude	Ability to model and embody mindful awareness (*Respond to participants in a curious, present-focused way, nonjudgmental/accepting of whatever arises*)	0	1	2	3	4
Theme	Integrates/refers to session theme throughout	0	1	2	3	4
Redirects/ Stays on topic	Redirects from content or "storytelling" to direct experience, keeps session on topic	0	1	2	3	4
Elicits	Elicits versus teaches themes	0	1	2	3	4
Clarifies intentions, disabuses expectations	Understands and clarifies intentions and addresses misconceptions about mindfulness or practice (*Addresses "I'm not doing it right" "It didn't work" "I'm in a totally different zone when I practice" "I'm trying but I can't seem to relax"*)	0	1	2	3	4

D. GLOBAL RATING

Overall quality of the therapy in this session				
Unsatisfactory	Mediocre	Satisfactory	Good	Excellent
0	1	2	3	4

References

Alexander, C. N., Robinson, P., Orme-Johnson, D. W., & Schneider, R. H. (1994). The effects of transcendental meditation compared to other methods of relaxation and meditation in reducing risk factors, morbidity, and mortality. *Homeostasis in Health and Disease, 35*(4–5), 243–263.

Amaro, H., Spear, S., Vallejo, Z., Conron, K., & Black, D. S. (2014). Feasibility, acceptability, and preliminary outcomes of a mindfulness-based relapse prevention intervention for culturally diverse, low-income women in substance use disorder treatment. *Substance Use and Misuse, 49*(5), 547–559.

American Psychiatric Association. (2013). *Diagnostic and statistical manual of mental disorders* (5th ed.). Arlington, VA: Author.

Barks, C. (Trans.). (1995). *The essential Rumi.* San Francisco: Harper.

Bellg, A., Borrelli, B., Resnick, B., Hecht, J., Sharp Minicucci, D., & Ory, M. (2004). Enhancing treatment fidelity in health behavior change studies: Best practices and recommendations from the NIH Behavior Change Consortium. *Health Psychology, 23,* 443–451.

Blume, A. W. (2016). Advances in substance abuse prevention and treatment interventions among racial, ethnic, and sexual minority populations. *Alcohol Research: Current Reviews, 38*(1), 47–54.

Blume, A. W., Lovato, L. V., Thyken, B. N., & Denny, N. (2012). The relationship of microaggressions with alcohol use and anxiety among ethnic minority college students in a historically White institution. *Cultural Diversity and Ethnic Minority Psychology, 18*(1), 45–54.

Bowen, S., Chawla, N., Collins, S., Witkiewitz, K., Hsu, S., Grow, J., . . . Marlatt, G. A. (2009). Mindfulness-based relapse prevention for substance use disorders: A pilot efficacy trial. *Substance Abuse, 30,* 295–305.

Bowen, S., Witkiewitz, K., Clifasefi, S. L., Grow, J., Chawla, N., Hsu, S. H., . . . Larimer, M. E. (2014). Relative efficacy of mindfulness-based relapse prevention, standard relapse prevention, and treatment as usual for substance use disorders: A randomized clinical trial. *JAMA Psychiatry, 71*(5), 547–556.

Bowen, S., Witkiewitz, K., Dillworth, T., Chawla, N., Simpson, T., Ostafin, B., . . . Marlatt, G. A. (2006). Mindfulness meditation and substance use in an incarcerated population. *Psychology of Addictive Behaviors, 20,* 343–347.

Brewer, J., Sinha, R., Chen, J. A., Michalsen, R. N., Babuscio, T. A., Nich, C., . . . Rounsaville, B. J. (2009). Mindfulness training and stress reactivity in substance abuse: Results from a randomized, controlled stage I pilot study. *Substance Abuse, 30,* 306–317.

Bureau of Justice Statistics, Office of Justice Programs, U.S. Department of Justice. (2018, January 9). *Prisoners in 2016* (NCJ 251149). Washington, DC: Author.

Chartier, K., & Caetano, R. (2010). Ethnicity and health disparities in alcohol research. *Alcohol Research and Health, 33*(1–2), 152–160.

Chawla, N., Collins, S., Bowen, S., Hsu, S., Grow, J., Douglas, A., & Marlatt, A. (2010). The Mindfulness-Based Relapse Prevention Adherence and Competence Scale: Development, interrater reliability, and validity. *Psychotherapy Research, 20*(4), 388–397.

Curado, D., Barros, V., Opaleye, E., Bowen, S., Hachul, H., & Noto, A. R. (2018). The role of mindfulness in the insomnia severity of female chronic hypnotic users. *International Journal of Behavioral Medicine, 25*(5), 526–531.

Curry, S., Marlatt, G. A., & Gordon, J. R. (1987). Abstinence violation effect: Validation of an attributional construct with smoking cessation. *Journal of Consulting and Clinical Psychology, 55,* 145–149.

Daley, D., & Marlatt, G. A. (2006). *Overcoming your drug or alcohol problem: Effective recovery strategies.* New York: Oxford University Press.

Davis, J. P., Barr, N., Dworkin, E. R., Dumas, T. M., Berey, B., DiGuiseppi, G., & Cahn, B. R. (2019). Effect of mindfulness-based relapse prevention on impulsivity trajectories among young adults in residential substance use disorder treatment. *Mindfulness, 10*(10), 1997–2009.

Donnenfield, D. (Producer/director). (1998). *Changing from inside* [DVD]. Onalaska, WA: Pariyatti.

Enkema, M. C., & Bowen, S. (2017). Mindfulness practice moderates the relationship between craving and substance use in a clinical sample. *Drug and Alcohol Dependence, 179,* 1–7.

Glasner, S., Mooney, L. J., Ang, A., Garneau, H. C., Hartwell, E., Brecht, M.-L., & Rawson, R. A. (2017). Mindfulness-based relapse prevention for stimulant dependent adults: A pilot randomized clinical trial. *Mindfulness, 8*(1), 126–135.

Greenfield, B. L., Roos, C., Hagler, K. J., Stein, E., Bowen, S., & Witkiewitz, K. A. (2018). Race/ethnicity and racial group composition moderate the effectiveness of mindfulness-based relapse prevention for substance use disorder. *Addictive Behaviors, 81,* 96–103.

Griffin, K. (2004). *One breath at a time: Buddhism and the twelve steps.* Emmaus, PA: Rodale.

Grow, J. (2013, November). *Effects of a pretreatment brief motivational intervention on treatment engagement in CBT-based and mindfulness-based relapse prevention.* Poster presented at the annual conference of the Association for Behavioral and Cognitive Therapies, Nashville, TN.

Guerrero, E. G. (2013). Enhancing access and duration in substance abuse treatment: The role of Medicaid payment acceptance and cultural competence. *Drug and Alcohol Dependence, 132,* 555–561.

Kabat-Zinn, J. (1990). *Full catastrophe living: Using the wisdom of your body and mind to face stress, pain, and illness.* New York: Delacorte.

Kabat-Zinn, J. (1994). *Wherever you go, there you are: Mindfulness meditation in everyday life.* New York: Hyperion.

Kabat-Zinn, J. (2002). *Guided mindfulness meditation* [CD recording]. Lexington, MA: Sounds True.

Kabat-Zinn, J. (2003). Mindfulness-based interventions in context: Past, present, and future. *Clinical Psychology Science and Practice, 10,* 144–156.

Killeen, T., Feigl, H., Shaw, M., & Bowen, S. (2018, June). *Perceptions of helpfulness of a mindfulness meditation program in women with PTSD and SUD.* Presentation at the 80th annual meeting of the College on Problems of Drug Dependence, San Diego, CA.

Lyons, T., Womack, V. Y., Cantrell, W. D., & Kenemore, T. (2019). Mindfulness-based relapse prevention in a jail drug treatment program. *Substance Use and Misuse, 54*(1), 57–64.

Marlatt, G. A. (2002). Buddhist philosophy and the treatment of addictive behavior. *Cognitive and Behavioral Practice, 9,* 44–50.

Marlatt, G. A., & Donovan, D. M. (Eds.). (2005). *Relapse prevention: Maintenance strategies in the treatment of addictive behaviors* (2nd ed.). New York: Guilford Press.

Marlatt, G. A., Pagano, R. R., Rose, R. M., & Marques, J. K. (1984). Effects of meditation and relaxation training upon alcohol use in male social drinkers. In D. H. Shapiro & R. N. Walsh (Eds.), *Meditation: Classic and contemporary perspectives* (pp. 105–120). New York: Aldine.

Marlatt, G. A., & Witkiewitz, K. (2005). Relapse prevention for alcohol and drug problems. In G. A. Marlatt & D. M. Donovan (Eds.), *Relapse prevention: Maintenance strategies in the treatment of addictive behaviors* (2nd ed., pp. 1–44). New York: Guilford Press.

Miller, W. R., & Rollnick, S. (2013). *Motivational Interviewing: Helping people change* (3rd ed). New York: Guilford Press.

Moyers, B. (1993). *Healing and the mind: Vol. 3. Healing from within* [Video recording]. New York: Public Broadcasting Service.

Murphy, T. J., Pagano, R. R., & Marlatt, G. A. (1986). Lifestyle modification with heavy alcohol drinkers: Effects of aerobic exercise and meditation. *Addictive Behaviors, 11*(2), 175–186.

O'Neill, R. E., Horner, R. H., Albin, R. W., Sprague, J. R., Storey, K., & Newton, J. S. (1997). *Functional assessment and program development for problem behavior: A practical handbook.* Pacific Grove, CA: Brooks/Cole.

Opaleye, E. S., Machado, M. P. A., Bowen, S., & Noto, A. R. (2019, October). *Feasibility of mindfulness-based relapse prevention to treatment for substance use disorders in Brazil: A mixed methods analyses.* Presented at the annual Mind and Life Europe Contemplative Science Symposium, Fürstenfeldbruck, Germany.

Powell, J. A. (2012). *Racing to justice: Transforming our conceptions of self and other to build an inclusive society.* Bloomington: Indiana University Press.

Roos, C., Bowen, S., & Witkiewitz, K. (in press). Approach coping and substance use outcomes following mindfulness-based relapse prevention among individuals with negative affect symptomatology. *Mindfulness.*

Roos, C. R., Kirouac, M., Stein, E., Wilson, A. D., Bowen, S., & Witkiewitz, K. (2018). An open trial of rolling admission mindfulness-based relapse prevention (rolling MBRP): Feasibility, acceptability, dose-response relations, and mechanisms. *Mindfulness, 10*(6), 1062–1073.

Segal, Z. V., Williams, J. M. G., & Teasdale, J. D. (2013). *Mindfulness-based cognitive therapy for depression* (2nd ed.). New York: Guilford Press.

Somohano, V., Manuel, J., Rutkie, R., & Bowen, S. (2016, June). *Mindfulness-based relapse prevention for clients in methadone maintenance treatment: A pilot feasibility trial.* Poster presentation at the Mind and Life Summer Research Institute, Garrison, NY.

Spicer, J. (1993). *The Minnesota model: The evolution of the multidisciplinary approach to addiction recovery.* Center City, MN: Hazelden.

Waltz, J., Addis, M., Koerner, K., & Jacobson, N. (1993). Testing the integrity of a psychotherapy protocol: Assessment of adherence and competence. *Journal of Consulting and Clinical Psychology, 61,* 620–630.

Witkiewitz, K., & Bowen, S. (2010). Depression, craving, and substance use following a randomized trial of mindfulness-based relapse prevention. *Journal of Consulting and Clinical Psychology, 78*(3), 362–374.

Witkiewitz, K., Bowen, S., Douglas, H., & Hsu, S. H. (2013). Mindfulness-based relapse prevention for substance craving. *Addictive Behaviors, 38*(2), 1563–1571.

Witkiewitz, K., Greenfield, B. L., & Bowen, S. (2013). Mindfulness-based relapse prevention with racial and ethnic minority women. *Addictive Behaviors, 38*(12), 2821–2824.

Witkiewitz, K., Warner, K., Sully, B., Barricks, A., Stauffer, C., Thompson, B. L., & Luoma, J. B. (2014). Randomized trial comparing mindfulness-based relapse prevention with relapse prevention for women offenders at a residential addiction treatment center. *Substance Use and Misuse, 49*(5), 536–546.

Index

Note. *f* or *t* following a page number indicates a figure or table.

A New Relationship with Discomfort (Session 2). *See* Session 2 (A New Relationship with Discomfort)

Abstinence, 19

Acceptance, 8, 19, 117–119, 126, 136–137. *See also* Session 5 (Acceptance and Skillful Action)

Acceptance and Skillful Action (Session 5). *See* Session 5 (Acceptance and Skillful Action)

Adapting the program. *See* Modified practices and adaptations to the program

Addiction and addictive behavior, 5–8, 172–173. *See also* Research on mindfulness and addiction

Agitation, 57–58, 71. *See also* Barriers to daily practice

Alcoholics Anonymous (AA), 18–20

Alternate formats to present material, 8, 27, 175–177. *See also* Modified practices and adaptations to the program; Sessions

Antecedents. *See* Triggers of addictive behaviors or relapse

Attendance, 21–22

Audio files. *See* Materials

Automatic pilot. *See also* Session 1 (Automatic Pilot and Mindful Awareness)
 Awareness of Hearing Exercise (Practice 3.1), 77
 inquiry and, 12
 overview, 30
 recognizing and interrupting, 8
 relapses and, 20, 133–137, 133*f*, 142
 SOBER Space Exercise (Practice 3.3), 83–84, 90–92

Automatic Pilot and Mindful Awareness (Session 1). *See* Session 1 (Automatic Pilot and Mindful Awareness)

Aversion, 54–56, 71. *See also* Barriers to daily practice

Awareness
 Awareness of Hearing Exercise (Practice 3.1), 76–78
 Body Scan Meditation (Practice 1.2), 41–43
 increasing, 8

 inquiry and, 10–12, 11*f*
 mindfulness of daily activity and, 44
 Raisin Exercise (Practice 1.1), 36–40
 Session 3 (From Reacting to Responding), 75

Awareness of Hearing Exercise (Practice 3.1), 76–78, 86, 187

Awareness of Seeing Exercise (Practice 4.1), 97, 104, 188

Barriers to daily practice, 21–22, 54–60, 71, 78–82. *See also* Daily practices

Body Scan Meditation (Practice 1.2), 41–43, 46–48, 185

Body Scan Meditation (Practice 8.1), 160, 164

Body scan meditations, 53–60, 78–82. *See also* Meditation practices

Breath Meditation (Practice 3.2), 82–83, 87–88, 187

Breath meditations, 82–84, 87–88, 90–92, 107–108. *See also* Meditation practices

Challenge zone of engagement, 26, 26*f*

Challenges. *See* Barriers to daily practice

Choice, 25, 133–137, 133*f*, 142

Clinician training and preparation, 1–2, 8, 13–18. *See also* Group facilitation

Closed enrollment format, 178–179

Co-facilitation, 13. *See also* Facilitation of a MBRP group

Compassion, 8, 19, 23, 146–147, 152–153

Concluding Meditation (Practice 8.2), 163, 165–166, 192

Contextual adaptations. *See* Modified practices and adaptations to the program

Coping skills, 19

Court mandated treatment, 21

Cravings. *See also* Barriers to daily practice; Session 1 (Automatic Pilot and Mindful Awareness); Urges
 daily practice and, 56–57
 False Refuge Exercise (Practice 3.3), 83, 89

Cravings (continued)
    mindfulness of daily activity and, 44
    overview, 63–64, 71
    Urge Surfing Exercise (Practice 2.2), 62–65, 64f,
        68–69
Cultural adaptations. See Modified practices and
    adaptations to the program

Daily activities
    mindfulness of, 44
    Session 3 (From Reacting to Responding), 76–78,
        85, 90–92
    Session 7 (Supporting and Sustaining Well-Being),
        147–149, 154
Daily practices. See also Barriers to daily practice;
    Meditation practices
    form for tracking, 51, 74, 85, 94, 111, 121, 127, 138,
        144, 156
    group facilitation and, 12–13
    introducing the idea of, 36
    maintaining a practice of beyond the course,
        161–163
    Session 1 (Automatic Pilot and Mindful
        Awareness), 36, 43–44, 50–51, 54–60
    Session 2 (A New Relationship with Discomfort),
        66, 73
    Session 3 (From Reacting to Responding), 84–85
    Session 4 (Mindfulness in Challenging Situations),
        97, 103
    Session 5 (Acceptance and Skillful Action), 121
    Session 6 (Seeing Thoughts as Thoughts), 131–132
    Session 7 (Supporting and Sustaining Well-Being),
        147, 151
    Session 8 (Social Support and Continuing
        Practice), 160
    supporting, 21–22
Desire, 56–57, 71. See also Barriers to daily practice
Diagnosis, 5–6
Direct experiences, 9–10, 11–12
Discomfort, 8, 55–56. See also A New Relationship
    with Discomfort (Session 2); Barriers to daily
    practice; Physical experiences
Distraction, 16. See also Barriers to daily practice
Doubt, 60, 71. See also Barriers to daily practice
Drowsiness, 58–60, 71. See also Barriers to daily
    practice

Economic inequalities, 6–7
Emotions, 16, 60–62
Engagement, zones of, 25–26, 26f
Extended session for mindfulness practice, 180

Facilitation of a MBRP group. See Group facilitation;
    Sessions; individual sessions
False Refuge Exercise (Practice 3.3), 83, 89, 187
Fidelity of implementation, 182–183, 193–194
Format, group, 20–23, 35–36, 177–182. See also
    Sessions
Forms. See Materials
Freedom, 19
Friendliness, 23, 146–147, 152–153
From Reacting to Responding (Session 3). See
    Session 3 (From Reacting to Responding)

Gender, 22
Goodwill, 146–147, 152–153
Group facilitation
    beginning and ending each session, 64
    co-facilitation, 13
    issues to consider, 23–27, 26f
    logistics involved in, 20–23, 35–36
    Mindfulness-Based Relapse Prevention–Fidelity
        Scale, 193–194
    overview, 8–13, 11f, 29
    12-step approaches, 18–20
Group structure and format, 20–23, 35–36, 177–182.
    See also Sessions

Habit/Comfort zone of engagement, 26, 26f
Habits, 12, 20, 44. See also Automatic pilot; Session 1
    (Automatic Pilot and Mindful Awareness)
HALT (Hungry, Angry, Lonely, Tired) acronym, 150
Handouts. See Materials
Harm reduction goals, 19
Home practice. See Daily practices; Meditation
    practices

Impulsive behaviors, 44, 62–65, 64f, 68–69. See
    also Session 1 (Automatic Pilot and Mindful
    Awareness)
Inquiry, 8, 9–12, 11f
In-session practices, 36. See also Meditation practices
Integrity of treatment, 182–183, 193–194

Kindness, 8, 23, 26, 146–147, 152–153
Kindness Meditation Exercise (Practice 7.1), 146–147,
    152–153, 191

Lapses
    discussing vulnerabilities to relapses, 149–150
    overview, 19–20
    relapse cycle and, 133–137, 133f, 142
    relapse risks and, 100–101
    Session 6 (Seeing Thoughts as Thoughts), 132
Legal issues, 21
Length of groups, 20–21, 180
Lovingkindness, 8, 23, 26, 146–147, 152–153
Lying down during practices, 24

Mandated treatment, 21
Materials
    audiovisual resources, 183–184
    Session 1 (Automatic Pilot and Mindful
        Awareness), 33–34, 43–44, 45–51
    Session 2 (A New Relationship with Discomfort),
        53, 66, 67–74
    Session 3 (From Reacting to Responding), 75, 78,
        80–82, 84–85, 86–94
    Session 4 (Mindfulness in Challenging Situations),
        95, 100–101, 103
    Session 5 (Acceptance and Skillful Action), 112
    Session 6 (Seeing Thoughts as Thoughts), 128,
        137–138, 139–144
    Session 7 (Supporting and Sustaining Well-Being),
        145, 147–149, 150–151, 152–157
    Session 8 (Social Support and Continuing
        Practice), 158, 161

Meditation practices. *See also* Daily practices; Modified practices and adaptations to the program; *individual exercises*
    extended session for mindfulness practice and, 180
    facilitators' personal mindfulness meditation practices and, 1–2, 8, 15–18
    inquiry and, 10
    intentions of, 185–192
    issues to consider, 23–27, 26*f*
    maintaining a practice of beyond the course, 161–163
    mindfulness of daily activity and, 44
    Mindfulness-Based Relapse Prevention–Fidelity Scale, 193–194
    Session 1 (Automatic Pilot and Mindful Awareness), 36–40, 41–43, 45, 46–48, 185
    Session 2 (A New Relationship with Discomfort), 26, 60–66, 64*f*, 67, 68–69, 71, 186
    Session 3 (From Reacting to Responding), 76–78, 82–84, 86, 87–88, 89, 90–92, 187
    Session 4 (Mindfulness in Challenging Situations), 97–100, 101–104, 105–106, 107–108, 109, 188
    Session 5 (Acceptance and Skillful Action), 114, 115–116, 122–123, 124–125, 189
    Session 6 (Seeing Thoughts as Thoughts), 129–131, 137, 139–140, 141, 190
    Session 7 (Supporting and Sustaining Well-Being), 146–147, 152–153, 191
    Session 8 (Social Support and Continuing Practice), 160, 163, 164, 165–166, 192
Metaphors, 176–177
Metta. *See* Lovingkindness
Mindfulness, 24–25, 40
Mindfulness in Challenging Situations (Session 4). *See* Session 4 (Mindfulness in Challenging Situations)
Mindfulness meditation practices. *See* Daily practices; Meditation practices
Mindfulness-based cognitive therapy (MBCT), 2
Mindfulness-based relapse prevention (MBRP) in general, 1–3, 18–23, 183–184, 193–194
Mindfulness-based stress reduction (MBSR), 2
Mindfulness-based treatments, 6–8. *See also* Research on mindfulness and addiction
Modified practices and adaptations to the program. *See also* Alternate formats to present material; Meditation practices
    alternative structures and formats, 176–182
    cultural adaptations, 175–177
    overview, 27
    research on MBRP and, 174–177
    technology and audiovisual resources, 183–184
    treatment integrity and, 182–183
    walking practices and, 103
Motivational issues, 21. *See also* Barriers to daily practice
Mountain Meditation (Practice 2.3), 65–66, 71, 186
Movement practices. *See also* Meditation practices
    mindful movement and, 120
    modified practices and, 27
    review of daily practices and, 131–132

Walking Down the Street Exercise (Practice 2.1), 60–62, 67, 186
Walking Meditation Exercise (Practice 4.4), 102–103, 109

Narcotics Anonymous (NA), 18–20

Open enrollment format, 178–179
Oppression, systems of, 6–8
Overwhelm zone of engagement, 26, 26*f*

Peace, 56–57. *See also* Barriers to daily practice
Physical experiences, 16, 27, 55–56, 60–62. *See also* Barriers to daily practice; Discomfort
Posttraumatic stress disorder (PTSD). *See* Trauma
Posture during practices, 24, 27, 120
Poverty, 6–7
Practice, daily. *See* Daily practices
Precourse meetings, 22–23
Privilege, 6–8

Racial inequalities, 6–7
Raisin Exercise (Practice 1.1), 36–40, 45, 185
Reactive behaviors. *See also* Session 1 (Automatic Pilot and Mindful Awareness); Session 3 (From Reacting to Responding)
    mindfulness of daily activity and, 44
    overview, 9–10
    relapse cycle and, 133–137, 133*f*, 142
    Urge Surfing Exercise (Practice 2.2), 62–65, 64*f*, 68–69
Relapse and relapse prevention
    discussing the importance of support networks, 160–161
    identifying triggers and vulnerabilities for, 149–150
    overview, 19–20
    relapse cycle and, 133–137, 133*f*, 142
    relapse risks and, 100–101
    Reminder Cards and, 150–151, 155
    Session 6 (Seeing Thoughts as Thoughts), 132
Relaxation, 56–57. *See also* Barriers to daily practice
Reminder Card, 150–151, 155
Research on mindfulness and addiction
    efficacy of meditation for treatment of addictive behavior, 172–173
    overview, 171–172
    research on MBRP, 173–177
    technology and audiovisual resources, 183–184
    treatment integrity and, 182–183
Restlessness, 57–58, 71. *See also* Barriers to daily practice
Rolling enrollment format, 178–179

Safety, 25–26, 26*f*
Seeing Thoughts as Thoughts (Session 6). *See* Session 6 (Seeing Thoughts as Thoughts)
Self-judgment, 23, 60, 131, 136–137. *See also* Barriers to daily practice
Sensory practices, 36–40, 76–78, 86, 97–100, 104

Session 1 (Automatic Pilot and Mindful Awareness).
        See also Sessions
    Body Scan Meditation (Practice 1.2), 41–43
    closing, 44
    daily practice following, 43–44, 54–60
    expectations and agreements and, 35
    intentions of, 185
    introducing mindfulness to group participants,
        40
    introductions, 35
    materials for, 33, 43–44, 45–51
    mindfulness of daily activity and, 44
    overview, 30, 33–34, 49
    Raisin Exercise (Practice 1.1), 36–40
Session 2 (A New Relationship with Discomfort). *See
        also* Sessions
    Body Scan Meditation (Practice 1.2), 53–54
    check-in, 53
    closing, 66
    home practice review and challenges, 54–60
    intentions of, 186
    materials for, 53, 66, 67–74
    Mountain Meditation (Practice 2.3), 65–66, 71
    overview, 30, 49, 52–53, 73
    Urge Surfing Exercise (Practice 2.2), 62–65, 64f,
        68–69
    Walking Down the Street Exercise (Practice 2.1),
        60–62, 67
Session 3 (From Reacting to Responding). *See also*
        Sessions
    Awareness of Hearing Exercise (Practice 3.1),
        76–78, 86
    Breath Meditation (Practice 3.2), 82–83, 87–88
    check-in, 76
    closing, 85
    daily practice and, 84–85
    False Refuge Exercise (Practice 3.3), 83, 89
    intentions of, 187
    materials for, 75, 84, 86–94
    overview, 30, 49, 75–76, 93
    review of daily practices, 78–82
    SOBER Space Exercise (Practice 3.3), 83–84,
        90–92
Session 4 (Mindfulness in Challenging Situations).
        See also Sessions
    Awareness of Seeing Exercise (Practice 4.1), 97,
        104
    check-in, 96–97
    closing, 103
    daily practice and, 103
    intentions of, 188
    materials for, 95, 103, 104–111
    overview, 30, 49, 95–96, 110
    relapse risks and, 100–101
    review of daily practices, 97
    Sitting Meditation: Sound, Breath, Sensation,
        Thought Exercise (Practice 4.2), 97–100,
        105–106
    SOBER Space in a Challenging Situation Exercise
        (Practice 4.3), 101–102, 107–108
    Walking Meditation Exercise (Practice 4.4),
        102–103, 109

Session 5 (Acceptance and Skillful Action). *See also*
        Sessions
    check-in, 114
    closing, 121
    daily practice and, 121
    discussing acceptance and skillful action and,
        117–119
    intentions of, 189
    materials for, 112, 117, 121, 122–127
    mindful movement and, 120
    overview, 30, 49, 112–113, 126
    review of daily practices, 114–115
    Sitting Meditation (Practice 5.1), 114, 122–123
    SOBER space and, 117
    SOBER Space (In Pairs) Exercise (Practice 5.2),
        115–116, 124–125
Session 6 (Seeing Thoughts as Thoughts). *See also*
        Sessions
    check-in, 129
    closing, 138
    daily practice and, 137–138
    intentions of, 190
    materials for, 128, 137–138, 139–144
    overview, 30, 49, 128–129, 143
    preparing for the end of the course and, 137–138
    relapse cycle and, 133–137, 133f, 142
    review of daily practices, 131–132
    Sitting Meditation: Thoughts Exercise (Practice
        6.1), 129–131, 139–140
    SOBER (*S*top, *O*bserve, *B*reath, *E*xpand, *R*espond)
        space and, 137
    SOBER Space Exercise (Practice 6.2), 137, 141
    thoughts and relapse and, 132
Session 7 (Supporting and Sustaining Well-Being).
        See also Sessions
    check-in, 146
    closing, 151
    Daily Activities Worksheet, 147–149, 154
    daily practice and, 151
    discussing vulnerabilities to relapses, 149–150
    intentions of, 191
    Kindness Meditation Exercise (Practice 7.1),
        146–147, 152–153
    materials for, 145, 147–149, 150–151, 152–157
    overview, 30, 49, 145–146, 156
    Reminder Cards, 150–151, 155
    review of daily practices and, 147
    SOBER space and, 150
Session 8 (Social Support and Continuing Practice).
        See also Sessions
    Body Scan Meditation (Practice 8.1), 160, 164
    check-in, 159
    closing circle, 163
    Concluding Meditation (Practice 8.2), 163, 165–166
    discussing the importance of support networks,
        160–161
    intentions of, 192
    maintaining a practice in the future, 161–163
    materials for, 158, 161, 164–169
    overview, 30, 49, 158–159, 169
    reflections on the course, 161, 168
    review of daily practices and, 160

Sessions. *See also* Alternate formats to present material; Facilitation of a MBRP group; Group facilitation; Group structure and format; *individual sessions*
  agenda for, 8
  alternative structures and formats, 177–182
  beginning and ending each session, 64
  intentions of, 185–192
  overview of, 29–30, 30*t*, 49
  six-week format for, 180–182
Sitting Meditation: Sound, Breath, Sensation, Thought, Emotion Exercise (Practice 5.1), 114, 122–123, 189
Sitting Meditation: Sound, Breath, Sensation, Thought Exercise (Practice 4.2), 97–100, 105–106, 188
Sitting Meditation: Thoughts Exercise (Practice 6.1), 129–131, 139–140, 190
Sitting posture during practices, 24, 27, 82–83, 84–85, 87–88, 131–132
Six-week format, 180–182
Size of groups, 22
Skillful action, 117–119, 126. *See also* Session 5 (Acceptance and Skillful Action)
Sleepiness, 58–60, 71. *See also* Barriers to daily practice
SOBER (*Stop, Observe, Breath, Expand, Respond*) space. *See also* Breath meditations
  form for tracking, 94, 111, 117, 125, 144, 156
  home practice and, 85
  materials for, 84, 90–92, 117, 121
  overview, 83–84, 93
  review of daily practices and, 114–115, 132
  Session 3 (From Reacting to Responding), 83–84, 90–92, 187
  Session 4 (Mindfulness in Challenging Situations), 101–102, 107–108, 188
  Session 5 (Acceptance and Skillful Action), 115–116, 124–125, 189
  Session 6 (Seeing Thoughts as Thoughts), 137, 141
  Session 7 (Supporting and Sustaining Well-Being), 150
SOBER Space Exercise (Practice 3.3), 83–84, 90–92, 187
SOBER Space Exercise (Practice 6.2), 137, 141
SOBER Space in a Challenging Situation Exercise (Practice 4.3), 101–102, 107–108, 188
SOBER Space (In Pairs) Exercise (Practice 5.2), 115–116, 124–125, 189
Social Support and Continuing Practice (Session 8). *See* Session 8 (Social Support and Continuing Practice)
Sociopolitical context of addiction, 6–8, 176

Structure of groups, 20–23, 35–36, 177–182. *See also* Sessions
Supporting and Sustaining Well-Being (Session 7). *See* Session 7 (Supporting and Sustaining Well-Being)

Technology, 183–184
Thoughts. *See also* Session 6 (Seeing Thoughts as Thoughts)
  facilitators' personal mindfulness meditation practices and, 16
  inquiry and, 9–10
  lovingkindness and, 23
  observing and labeling, 130–131
  relapse cycle and, 133–137, 133*f*, 142
  Sitting Meditation: Thoughts Exercise (Practice 6.1), 129–131
  Walking Down the Street Exercise (Practice 2.1), 60–62
Timing of groups, 20–21
Training. *See* Clinician training and preparation
Transcendental Meditation (TM), 172
Trauma, 25–26, 26*f*, 175
Treatment integrity, 182–183
Triggers of addictive behaviors or relapse
  discussing vulnerabilities to relapses, 149–150
  form for tracking, 72, 80–82, 100–101
  overview, 149–150
  relapse and, 100–101, 133–137, 133*f*, 142
  Session 2 (A New Relationship with Discomfort), 66, 72
  Session 4 (Mindfulness in Challenging Situations), 101–102
  12-step approaches, 19
12-step approaches, 18–20

Urge surfing, 26, 63–65, 64*f*, 101–102, 176–177
Urge Surfing Exercise (Practice 2.2), 26, 62–65, 64*f*, 68–69, 186
Urges, 44, 60–62, 63–65, 64*f*. *See also* Cravings; Session 1 (Automatic Pilot and Mindful Awareness)

Walking Down the Street Exercise (Practice 2.1), 60–62, 67, 186
Walking Meditation Exercise (Practice 4.4), 102–103, 109, 188
Wanting. *See* Cravings; Desire
Worksheets. *See* Materials

Younger clients, 27

Zones of engagement, 25–26, 26*f*

List of Audio Tracks

Track	Title	Run time
Session 1		
1	Body Scan	23:19
Session 2		
2	Urge Surfing	6:00
3	Mountain Meditation	9:38
Session 3		
4	Sitting Meditation (Breath)	15:55
5	SOBER Space	3:20
Session 5		
6	Sitting Meditation (Sound, Breath, Sensation, Thought, Emotion)	9:43
7	Mindful Movement	15:42
Session 6		
8	Sitting Meditation (Thoughts)	11:41
Session 7		
9	Kindness Meditation	16:29

Tipping With

Origami Money Folds

A novel and easy way of showing your appreciation of good service

Arnold Tubis

To Charlotte

Front cover photo $6 Tip

Back cover photo $1 Tip #3

Origami models designed and folded by Arnold Tubis.

Photography and folding steps by Arnold Tubis

Cover design by createspace.com.

Copyright

Copyright © 2013 by Arnold Tubis

Please send comments, suggested corrections and clarifications, and requests for assistance in making the money folds in this book to Arnold Tubis (tubisa@aol.com).

Manufactured in the United States of America by CreateSpace.com (www.createspace.com).

International Standard Book Number

ISBN-13:9780615867649(Arnold Tubis)

ISBN-10:0615867642

Table of Contents

Page

Introduction   4

Origami Folding Symbols   5

Some Basic Folding Maneuvers – Rabbit ears and Squashes   6

$1 Tip #1 George Washington Crossing the Delaware   7

$1 Tip #2   10

$1 Tip #3   12

$1 Tip #4   14

$2 Tip #1   16

$2 Tip #2   18

$2 Tip #3   20

$2 Tip #4 George Washington in a Ninja-Star Frame   22

$3 Tip #1   26

$3 Tip #2   29

$4 Tip   George Washington in a Star-of-David Frame   32

$6 Tip   Hexagonal Star   36

About the author   39

Introduction

Tipping for services well done is a long-standing tradition. Although we frequently tip these days via credit or debit cards, giving money directly still reflects a more personal and gracious old world manner of showing appreciation.

It is tempting to try to give as tips some of the elegant money fold designs of animals, birds, and sea life of origami artists such as Stephen Weiss, John Montroll, and Won Park. However, it is somewhat challenging to remember how to fold them (and to fold them well) especially when they are needed in a hurry on random occasions. This book shows how you can, with simple or low-intermediate folding skills and some practice, learn to fold a dozen different tips from dollar bills – tips that have attractive attention-grabbing geometric designs and prominently display the face (or faces) of George Washington. The identical pieces that make up three of the $2 tips also make presentable $1 tips. For each money fold, large and clear photographic details precede the folding steps.

Mathematically minded readers will recognize in the folding steps some well known methods of constructing angles of measures 22.5^0, 30^0, 45^0, 60^0, and 90^0, as well as squares, equilateral triangles, regular hexagons, and six-pointed stars. Math teachers and their students might therefore find these money folds to be useful in the classroom or for special studies and projects. It is an interesting coincidence that the square root of three, which is important in the geometry of equilateral triangles, is equal to 1.732..., and that George Washington was born in 1732.

Fresh new dollar bills will greatly enhance the appearance of the tips and the appreciation of their recipients. For practice, and/or classroom purposes, realistic fake bills are readily available from several online sources. (See, e.g., www.banksupplies.com). The $6 tip shown in the photos on page 36 was made from fake bills.

I have taught these tips at several meetings of the Greater San Diego Origami Group, and thank the members for their critiques of the folding steps.

I designed most of these money folds while sitting with my loving wife, Charlotte, during the seemingly endless hours of her treatment at the University of California San Diego Medical Center in La Jolla. I dedicate this book to her.

I also wish to thank Patsy Wang-Iverson of the Gabriela and Paul Rosenbaum Foundation and Origami USA for encouraging and promoting my money fold design efforts.

Arnold Tubis
Carlsbad, CA
November, 2013

Origami Folding Symbols

The symbols below are used throughout this book. Refer to this list whenever you are unsure of a symbol's meaning.

Symbol	Meaning	Symbol	Meaning
	Fold in the direction of the arrow.		Fold and unfold.
	Make a valley fold in the direction of the arrow. The arrow will sometimes not be shown.		A completed valley fold.
	Make a mountain fold. (Fold to the back.) The arrow will usually not be shown.		A completed mountain fold.
	A previously folded crease line.		Place your finger(s) here.
	Width of rectangle divided in half.		Bisected angle.

Some Basic Folding Maneuvers – Rabbit Ears and Squashes

The most difficult steps for novices in this book will probably be those for the formation of a so-called *rabbit ear* flap, followed in most cases by the symmetric squashing of the flap. We outline the folding sequences below.

After folding crease lines such as those in (a), simultaneously fold along these lines according to the mountain/valley fold designations in (b) to obtain a *rabbit ear* flap shown in (c). If then required, make an angle-bisecting fold as in (d), and then insert your finger into the flap and squash it symmetrically as in (e) to obtain the configuration in (f).

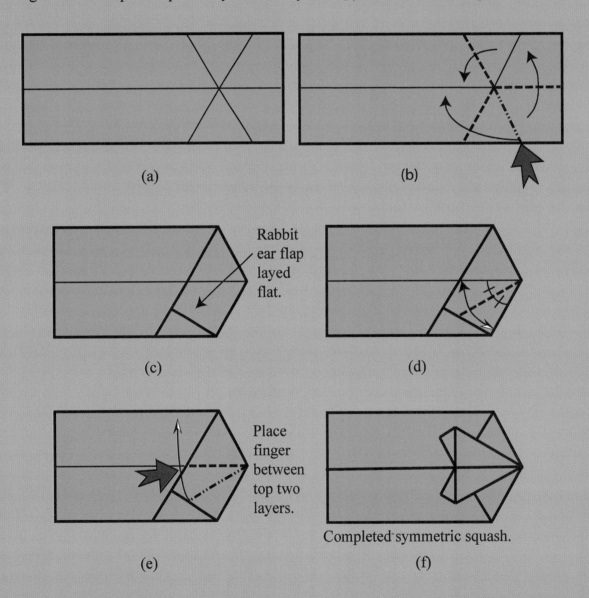

(a)

(b)

Rabbit ear flap layed flat.

(c)

(d)

Place finger between top two layers.

(e)

Completed symmetric squash.

(f)

$1 Tip #1 George - Washington Crossing the Delaware

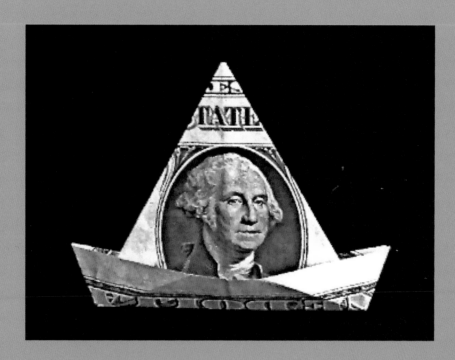

This model was inspired by the money fold, *Crossing the Delaware*, by the late Cyril Tessier.

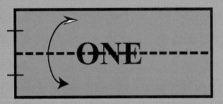

1. Start with back of bill facing up. Valley fold/unfold width in half.

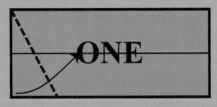

2. Valley fold so as to obtain the configuration of the piece in step 3.

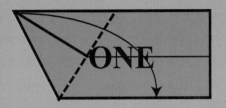

3. Valley fold.

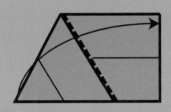

4. Valley fold.

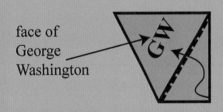

face of George Washington

5. Valley fold and tuck flap into pocket. to form an equilateral (60-60-60) triangle.

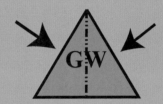

6. Push in sides, form mountain folds on front and back, and symmetrically pinch to the form shown in step 7.

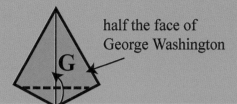

half the face of
George Washington

7. Valley fold up in front and back.

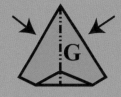

8. Push in sides, form mountain folds on
front and back, and pinch back to the
the form shown in step 9.

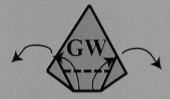

9. Pull out and valley fold up on both sides
so that a boat is formed under George
Washington.

10. George Washington
Crossing the Delaware.

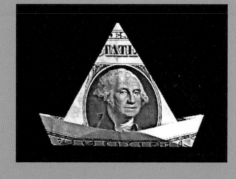

$1 Tip #2

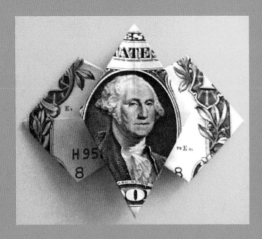

Front view

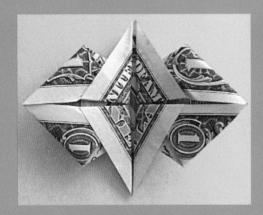

Back view

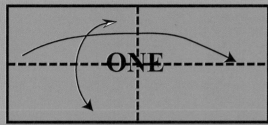

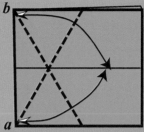

1. Valley fold/unfold in half vertically. Then valley fold in half horizontally.

2. Bring point *a* to the midline and valley fold/unfold. Do likewise with point *b*. Then unfold.

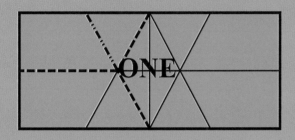

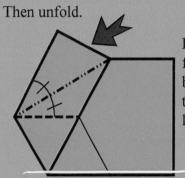

Place finger between top two layers.

3. Make a rabbit ear and lay it flat. (See page 6.)

4. Lift up the rabbit ear and symmetrically squash it. (See page 6.)

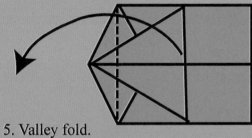

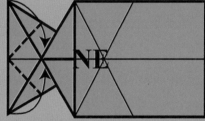

See photo of finished piece on page 10.

5. Valley fold.

6. Make valley folds and tuck flaps into pockets. Repeat steps 3-6 on the right side. Then turn over to view GW's face.

$1 Tip #3

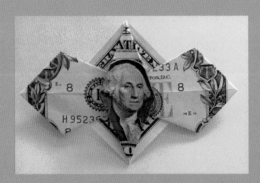

Front view

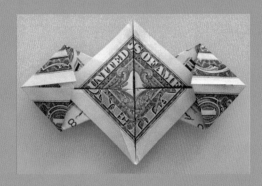

Back view

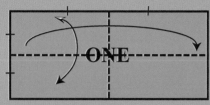

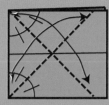

1. Valley fold/unfold in half vertically. Then valley fold in half horizontally.

2. Make valley fold/unfold creases as indicated.

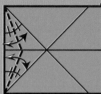

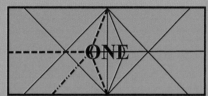

3. Make valley fold/unfold creases as indicated. Then completely unfold.

4. Make rabbit ear and then lay it flat as shown on page 6.

Insert finger between top two layers.

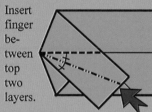

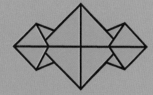

5. Lift up and symmetrically squash rabbit ear as shown on page 6.

6. Valley fold.

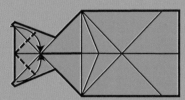

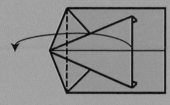

7. Make indicated valley folds, and then repeat steps 4 - 7 on the right side.

8. Turn over to show the face of George Washington.

$1 Tip #4

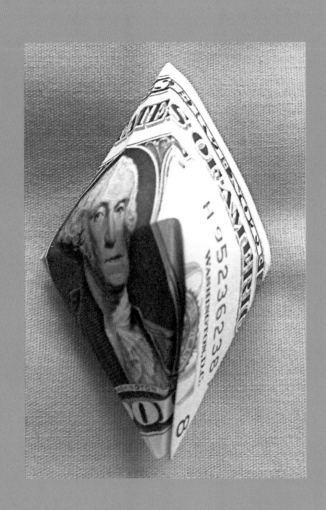

3-D Ornament

$1 Tip #4

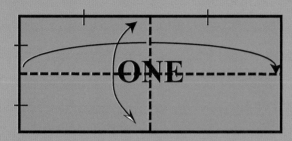

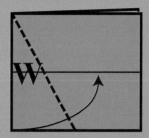

1. Valley fold/unfold in half vertically, and then valley fold in half horizontally.

2. Valley fold so as to get the configuration in step 3.

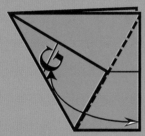

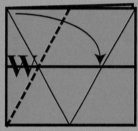

3. Valley fold/unfold, and then unfold to the configuraion in step 4.

4. Valley fold so as to get the configuration in step 5.

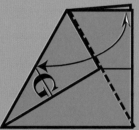

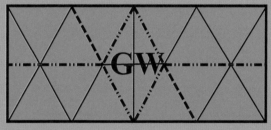

5. Valley fold/unfold, and then unfold completely.

6. Simultaneously form the six mountain and two valley folds.

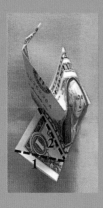

7. In succession, make valley folds **1** and **2**, and insert the resulting folded tab into the slit located along valley fold line **2**. Repeat the same operations with the upper tab.

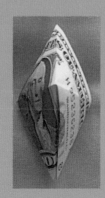

8. The completed model showing its 3-D ornamental aspect.

$2 Tip #1

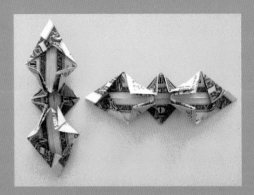

Before assembly

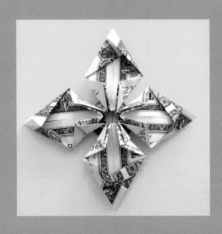

Asssembled (back view)

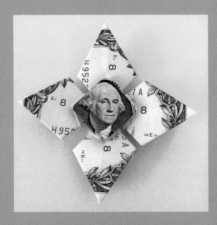

Front view

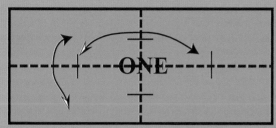 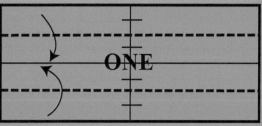

1. Valley fold/unfold in half vertically and horizontally.

2. Make valley folds so that the width of the piece is halved.

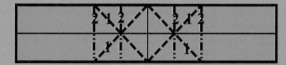 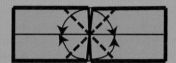

3. On left and right sides of the piece, form valley fold/unfold pairs **1** and mountain fold pairs **2**. Then collapse the piece on both sides to the configuration in step 4.

4. Make the four indicated valley folds.

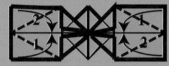 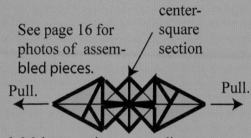

5. In succession, make valley fold pairs **1** and **2**.

See page 16 for photos of assembled pieces.

center-square section

Pull.   Pull.

6. Make two pieces according to steps 1 - 5. Pull open the small center-square sections of each, and insert one into the other so that the long axes of the pieces are perpendicular to each other. Press flat and turn over to view GW.

$2 Tip #2

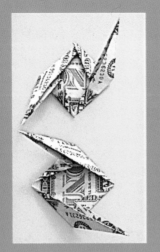

Single units can be used as $1 tips.

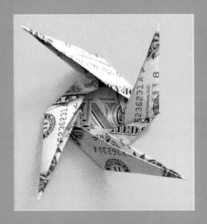

Before assembly

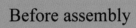

Assembled (back view)

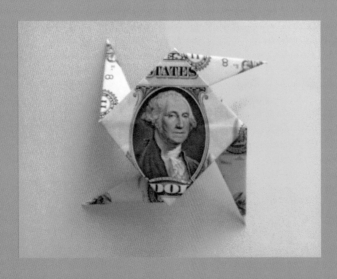

Front view

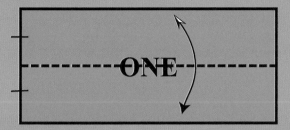

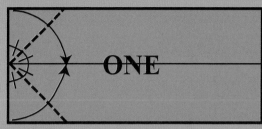

1. Valley fold/unfold in half vertically.

2. Make valley folds so as to obtain the configuration in step 3.

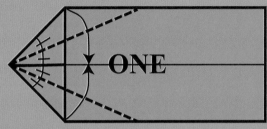

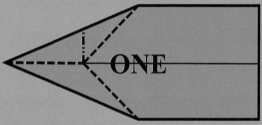

3. Make valley folds so as to obtain the configuration in step 4.

4. Make rabbit-ear flap and lay it flat as described on page 6.

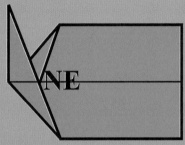

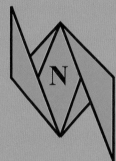

5. Repeat steps similar to 2 - 4 on the right side, with the resulting flap pointing down.

6. Make another piece according to steps 1-5, assemble them (see page 18), and then turn the piece over to show the face of GW.

$2 Tip #3

Single units can be used as $1 tips.

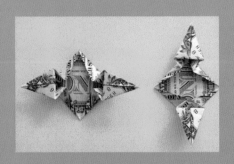

Before assembly

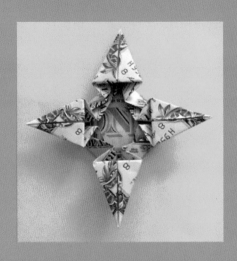

Assembled (back view)

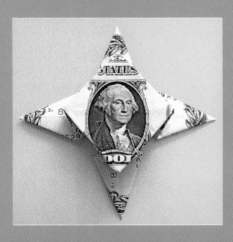

Front view

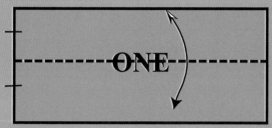

1. Valley fold/unfold in half vertically.

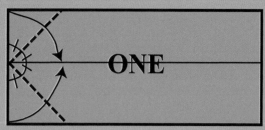

2. Make valley folds so as to obtain the configuration in step 3.

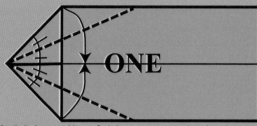

3. Make valley folds so as to obtain the configuration in step 4.

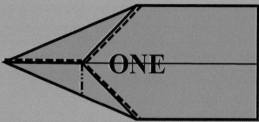

4. Form a rabbit ear flap and then squash it symmetrically, as described on page 6.

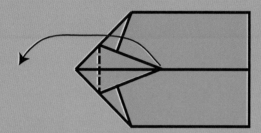

5. Valley fold, and then repeat steps 2-5 on the right side.

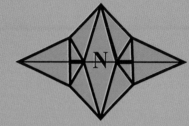

6. Fold another identical piece, and assemble. (See page 20.) Then turn piece over to show the face of GW.

$2 Tip #4 - George Washington in a Ninja-Star Frame

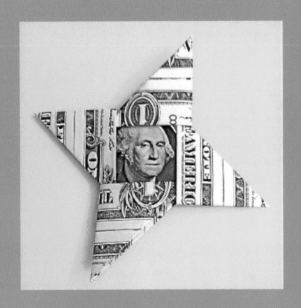

Front view

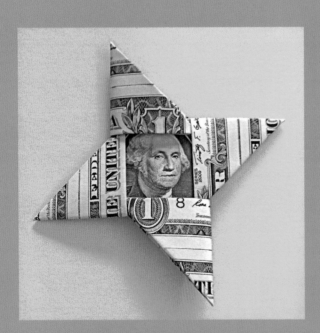

Back view

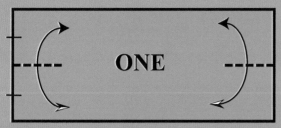

1. Make the pinch creases on the left and right.

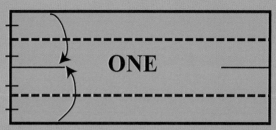

2. Valley fold raw side edges to the center crease. Then turn the piece over.

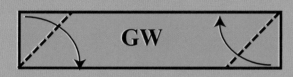

3. Make the two indicated valley folds.

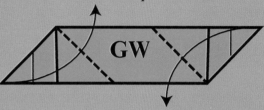

4. Make two more valley folds.

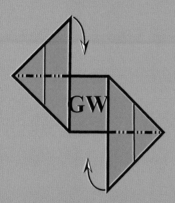

5. Make the indicated mountain folds. Then unfold.

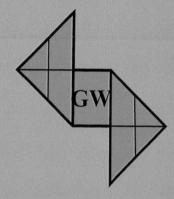

6. The folding of bill #1 is now complete.

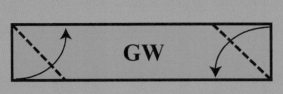 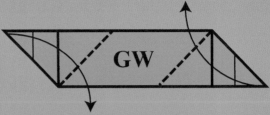

7. Start folding another bill using steps 1 and 2. Then make the two valley folds.

8. Make the indicated valley folds.

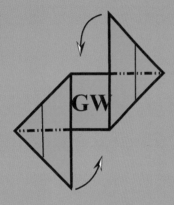 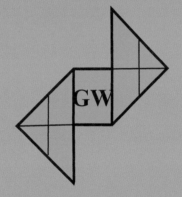

9. Make the indicated mountain folds. Then unfold.

10. The folding of bill #2 is now complete.

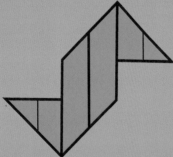 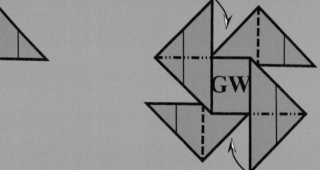

11. Turn piece from step 10 over and orient it like this. Place bill from step 6 over it as shown in step 12.

12. Make indicated mountain and valley folds. Tuck tips of the four folded flaps into the four pockets that are formed. (See steps 13 and 14.)

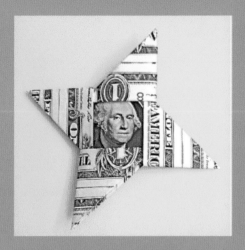

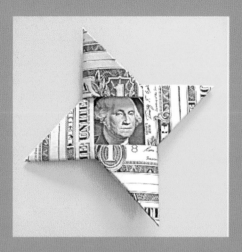

13. Top view of piece in step 12 after completion of the folding.

14. View of the underside of the piece In step 12 after completion of the folding.

Folding Hints

Note that on the top face of the configuration in step 12, each of the two mountain folds establishes a pocket into which the tip of the flap from a valley fold slides and thus forms a lock. (See step 13.) After completion of the mountain and valley folds on the top face, turn the piece over and slip the remaining loosed flaps tips into pockets that are already formed. (See step 14.) For extensive photographic detail about the folding of a standard Ninja Star (without frames), that shows the locking of the flaps, see, e.g., www.wikihow.com/Fold-an-Origami-Star-(Shuriken).

$3 Tip #1

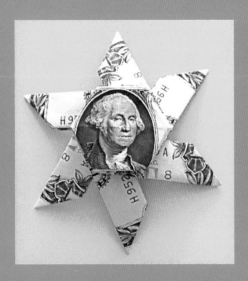

Front view

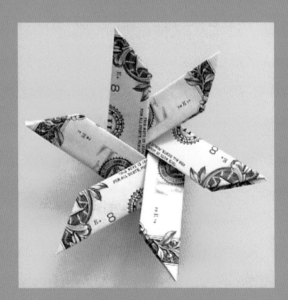

Back view

$3 Tip #1

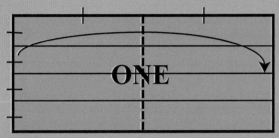

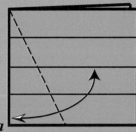

1. Fold in quarters vertically and valley fold in half horizontally.

2. Bring point *a* to the central horizontal line and valley fold/unfold.

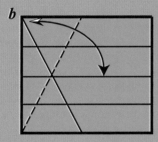

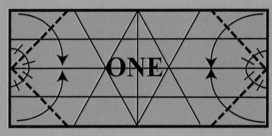

3. Bring point *b* to the central horizontal line and valley fold/unfold. Then unfold completely.

4. Make the four indicated valley folds.

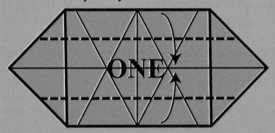

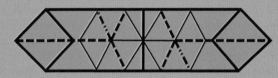

5. Make the two valley folds.

6. Form two rabbit ear flaps and lay them flat as shown on page 6.

7. Make two more pieces following steps 1 - 6.

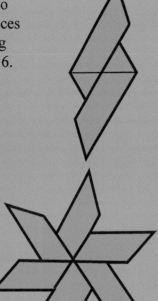

8. Slightly loosen the flaps of one piece and slip another piece into it as shown.

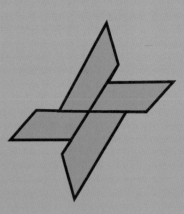

9. Slightly loosen the flaps of the third piece and slip the piece of step 8 into it.

10. Turn the piece over to show the face of George Washing - ton.

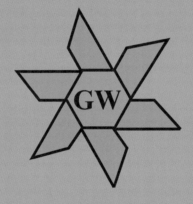

$3 Tip #2

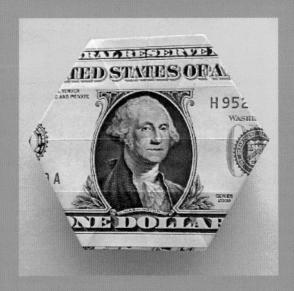

Front view

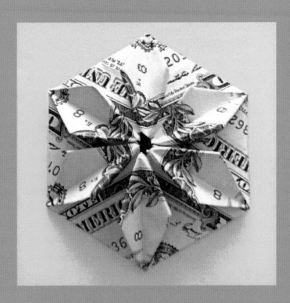

Back view

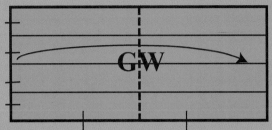

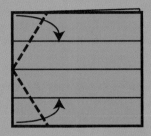

1. Fold the bill vertically in quarters, and then valley fold in half horizontally.

2. Make valley folds so as to obtain the configuration of the piece in step 3.

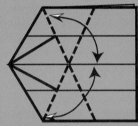

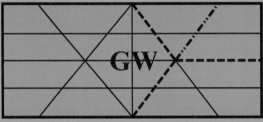

3. Make the two valley fold/unfold creases and then completely unfold.

4. Form a rabbit ear and lay it flat as shown on page 6.

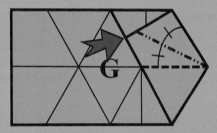

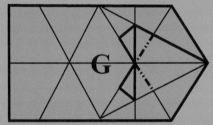

5. Lift up the rabbit ear and symmetrically squash it as shown on page 6. Some horizontal crease lines are not shown.

6. Make the two mountain folds on the top two layers. These folds should be *on top of* (i.e., not straddle) the third layer.

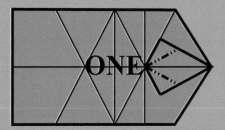 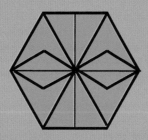

7. Make the two mountain folds. Then repeat steps 4 - 7 on the left side.

8. Fold two more identical pieces following steps 1 - 7.

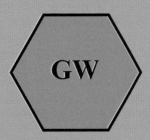

9. Slip one piece into the other.

10. Slip the piece in step 9 into a third one.

GW

Opposite side, showing face of George Washington.

$4 Tip - George Washington in a Star-of-David Frame

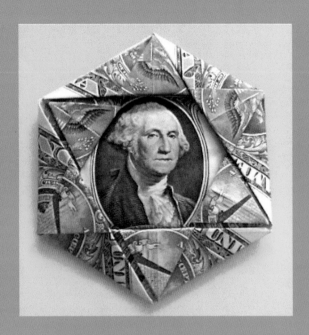

Front view

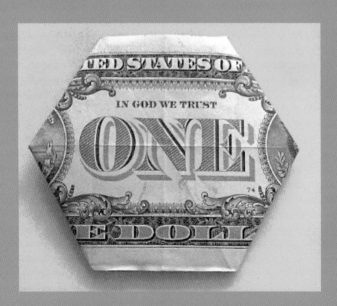

Back view

$4 Tip

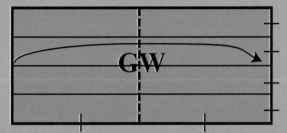

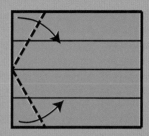

1. Valley fold/unfold a bill vertically in quarters, and then valley fold in half horizontally.

2. Make valley folds so as to obtain the configuration of the piece in step 3.

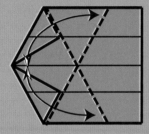

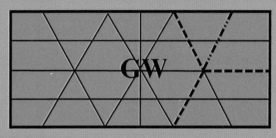

3. Make the two valley fold/unfold creases and then completely unfold.

4. Form a rabbit ear and lay it flat as shown on page 6.

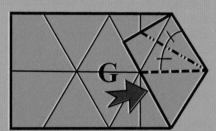

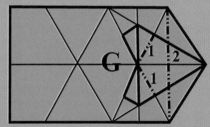

5. Lift up rabbit ear and symmetrically squash it as shown on page 6.

6. Make mountain folds **1** on the top two layers and then make mountain fold **2** so as to form a triangular pocket.

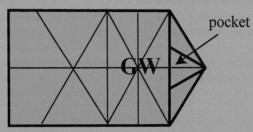

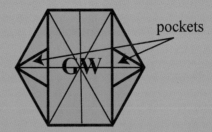

7. Repeat steps 4-6 on the left side so that two triangular pockets are formed.

8. Make three identical pieces using steps 1-7.

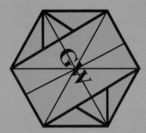

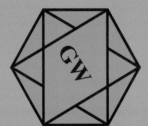

Some crease lines are not shown.

9. Orient one of the pieces like this and slip it into the piece in step 8, as shown in step 10.

10. Rotate the combined piece so that GW's head is pointed southeast and insert it into a third piece oriented as in step 8.

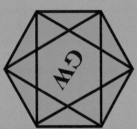

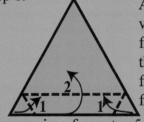

Adjust valley folds so that piece fits into frame.

11. The hexagonal Star-of-David frame is now complete.

12. Turn over piece from step 5 of *George Washington Crossing the Delaware.* In succession, make valley folds **1** and **2**.

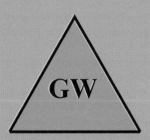

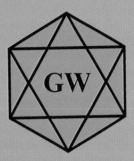

13. Turn over the piece in step 12 and insert into the frame in step 11.

14. George Washington in a Star-of-David frame.

Learning how to fold this model well will require some practice, and I recommend that you use fake bills before working with real ones. Poking into the pockets and making them as roomy as possible with a pointed bone folder in steps 6 and 7 will help in achieving good fits when putting the pieces together to form the frame in steps 9-11.

$6 Tip – Hexagonal Star

These stars were made with fake $1 bills.

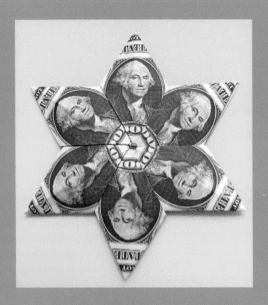

Front view

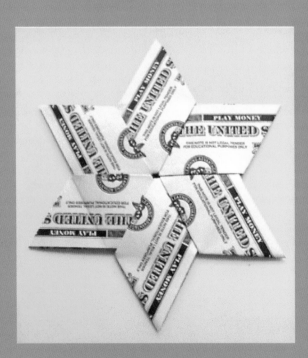

Back view

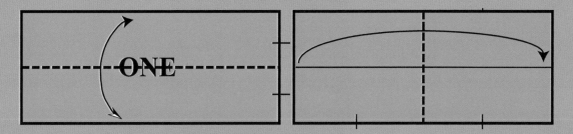

1. Valley fold/unfold vertically in half.   2. Valley fold the length in half.

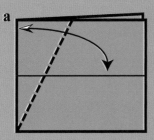

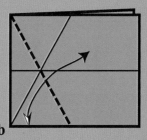

3. Bring point a to the horizontal center
line and valley fold/unfold.

4. Bring point **b** to the horizontal center
line and valley fold/unfold. Then completely unfold.

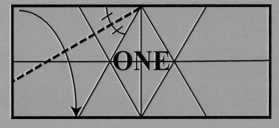

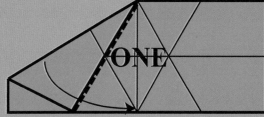

5. Valley fold.   6. Valley fold.

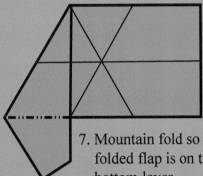

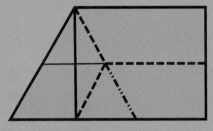

7. Mountain fold so that the folded flap is on top of the bottom layer.

8. Make a rabbit ear flap and lay it flat as described on page 6.

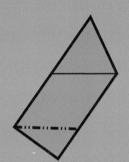

9. Mountain fold and tuck flap into the pocket underneath.

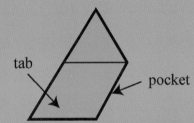

tab

pocket

10. Fold five more identical pieces according to steps 1 - 9. Then join them together as a star by tucking the tab on the lower left of one into the pocket on the lower right of the neighboring one. Turn the star over to show the six faces of George Washington.

See photos on page 36.

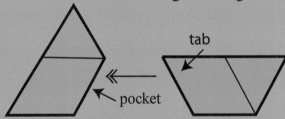

tab

pocket

About the Author

Arnold Tubis is a retired physics professor who was a faculty member at Purdue University in West Lafayette, Indiana from 1960 to 2000 (9 years as department head). He now lives in Carlsbad, California. Origami has been an avocation of his since the early 1960s and his models have been exhibited in the USA, Japan, Europe, and Israel. He is the co-author of *Decorative Origami Boxes from Single Squares* (with Leon Brown, British Origami Society, 2003), *Unfolding Mathematics with Origami Boxes* (with Crystal Elaine Mills, Key Curriculum Press, 2006), and *Fun with Folded Fabric Boxes* (with Crystal Elaine Mills, C&T Publications, 2007). He has also authored or co-authored about 15 papers on origami in K-12 mathematics education. He is currently focused on designing models that require, at most, a low-intermediate folding skill level, and can be used to enrich the teaching of geometry in middle school and high school. He is currently the coordinator of the Greater San Diego Origami Group.

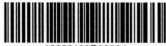

Printed in Great Britain
by Amazon.co.uk, Ltd.,
Marston Gate.

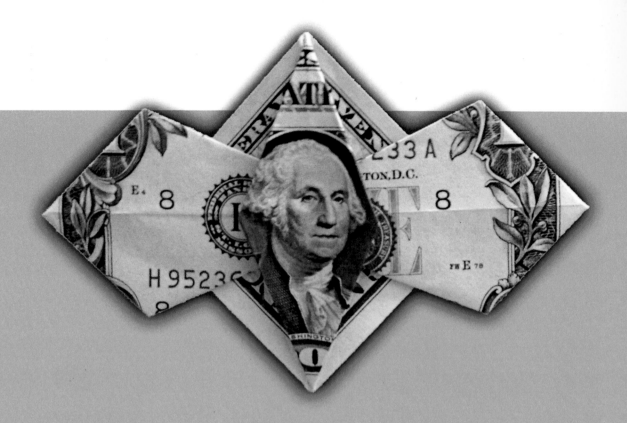

Practice, in a novel way, the time-honored tradition of giving tips for good service by learning how to make a dozen origami money folds with eye-catching geometric designs. By following the clear folding steps (including photographic detail), you should be able to fold all or most of the tips (involving one, two, three, four or six dollar bills) in a reasonably short time. Fresh, new dollar bills will greatly improve the appearance of the folded tips and increase the pleasure of their recipients.

ISBN 978-0-9815297-6

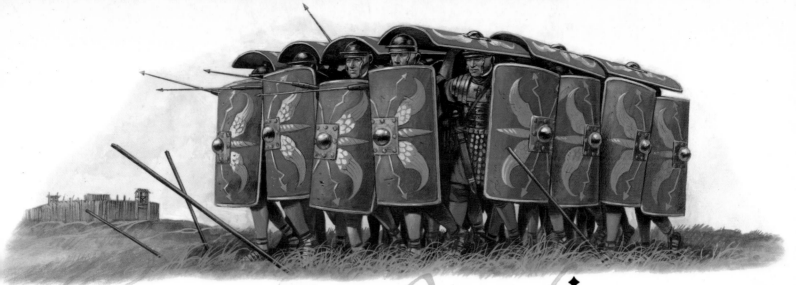

ENCYCLOPEDIA OF
BRITISH
HISTORY

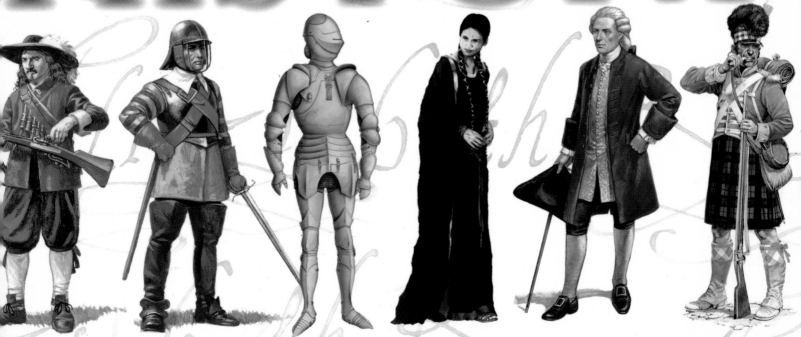

From prehistory to the present day